DISEASES AND PARASITES OF SHEEP & GOATS

DISEASES AND PARASITES OF SHEEP & GOATS

Editor
Gove Hambidge

BIOTECH
2026
Biotech Books

ISBN10 81-7622-087-6
ISBN13 978-81-7622-087-3

Published by : **BIOTECH BOOKS**
7462-63/23, Ansari Road, Darya Ganj,
New Delhi - 110002
Phones : 011 4300 3222
Email : biotechbooks@yahoo.co.in

PRINTED IN INDIA

CONTENTS

INTRODUCTION

Foot Rot of Sheep

Foot rot is sometimes a major disease of sheep (and occasionally of goats), especially where crowded corrals oı pastures are used. It is caused by infection of the hoofs, though authorities do not yet agree on the specific organism involved; several different micro-organisms have been found to be associated with the disease. Starting with lameness, redness, swelling, and intense pain around the hoofs, the symptoms may progress until even the bones and joints become involved. Sometimes animals seem to recover spontaneously, but the infection remains.

The treatment described by Shahan is effective but should be carried out by a veterinarian. It consists in (1) segregating all animals showing symptoms; (2) carefully trimming the hoofs and cutting away all dead tissue; (3) disinfecting the feet with a suitable antiseptic, usually copper sulphate (blue stone), which must be handled with caution. For a few sheep, a bucket may be used for dipping the feet; large numbers are usually driven through a shallow trough containing the antiseptic. The nature and strength of the antiseptic and the length of time the sheep should stand in it depend on the severity of the disease.

Prevention, of course, is better than cure. Shahan advises such measures as (1) quarantining newly purchased sheep for at least a month; (2) perhaps selling all infected sheep for slaughter under inspection instead of treating them; (3) thoroughly cleaning and disinfecting barns, sheds, corrals, etc., used by infected sheep; (4) taking special precautions after handling infected sheep; (5) draining muddy corrals and wet pastures if possible;. (6) removing healthy sheep to fresh ground and keeping them off infected pastures for 1 to 4 months, depending on the location and season.

Sore Mouth of Sheep and Goats

A highly contagious disease caused by a virus, sore mouth usually attacks animals less than a year old, producing raw sores, chiefly around the mouth. Occasionally older animals are infected, and the sores may appear elsewhere, notably on the udders of nursing dams. Subsequent bacterial infection may occur, with a high mortality, or the sores may become infested with screwworms. The chief damage from uncomplicated sore mouth comes from serious interference with feeding, which causes loss of weight and failure to grow. The disease is also known as contagious ecthyma.

Within recent years an effective vaccine has been developed. Applied much like smallpox vaccine, it confers immunity for several months to 2 years or longer. In range areas were the disease is known to prevail, vaccination may be done at the time of marking; in the case of feed-lot sheep, it should be done at least 10 days before the animals are shipped. As Shahan points out, it should be left to the veterinarian to decide whether vaccination should be used in any given case, or whether isolation of affected animals and disinfection of the premises are sufficient. Medicinal aid is seldom required and is rarely practical; the chief aim, after a case occurs, should be to prevent bacterial and screwworm infections.

Miscellaneous Diseases of Sheep and Goats

Shahan discusses some 36 or more diseases and injuries that affect sheep and goats, for the most part those not discussed elsewhere. They can be little more than mentioned in this brief summary. Many of them are largely preventable by good management, especially sanitation.

Diseases of the Digestive Organs

1. Bloat, an accumulation of gas in the stomach or intestines, resulting from the consumption of damaged or unsuitable feeds, is dangerous in an acute form and must then be treated practically by first-aid methods.
2. Constipation resulting from impaction of foodstuffs can be relieved by drugs, water, laxatives, and manipulation.

3. Diarrhoea may be due to any one of many different causes, discussed under other diseases.
4. Enterotoxemia, or intestinal poisoning, probably the most frequent cause of losses of lambs in western feed lots, results from the overeating of concentrates or lush forage. Prevention is a matter of good management; treatment is seldom successful.

Diseases of the Respiratory System

5. Hemorrhagic septicemia, or shipping fever, attacks sheep and goats as well as cattle. It is discussed briefly by Shahan and at length elsewhere in this volume.
6. Nasal catarrh, or snuffles, is common in sheep but seldom serious unless it is a symptom of some severe disease, in which case control and treatment depend on the cause.

Diseases of the Nervous System

7. Listerellosis, or circling disease, is a severe, incurable, usually fatal inflammation of the brain caused by infection with *Listerella* organisms.
8. Rabies, discussed elsewhere in this volume, is brought to sheep and goats, as to other animals, by the bites of rabid dogs.
9. Meningitis, an inflammation of the lining membranes (meninges) of the central nervous system, may be produced in sheep by infection with any one of several micro-organisms, including *Staphylococci* and *Streptococci*. Treatment is almost never practical.
10. Paralysis is usually an accompaniment of one of the infections of the central nervous system, but it may sometimes be due to the bites of certain ticks or to injuries to the spine.

Diseases of the Skin

11. Purulent dermatitis is due to invasion of the skin by pus-forming micro-organisms that enter through injuries or wounds. In severe cases, general poisoning of the system may result.

12. Ringworm, caused by various fungi, is relatively rare in sheep.
13. Sheep pox, which is similar to but not identical with smallpox in man, has not become established in the United States.
14. Actinobacillosis, an infectious disease caused by micro-organisms that enter through small punctures or cuts, is discussed at length elsewhere in the Yearbook under Miscellaneous Diseases of Cattle.

Diseases Connected with Reproduction

15. Abortion in sheep is rarely due to *Brucella* organisms, but it may be caused by any one of several other infections as well as by damaged feeds, injury, under-nourishment, and various diseases. Goats may contract brucellosis or other infections causing abortion.
16. Pregnancy toxemia includes pregnancy disease of sheep and also milk fever. Both are discussed elsewhere in the Yearbook, the latter under the diseases of cattle.
17. Metritis is an inflammation of the uterus due to any one of various infections. It is associated with abortion or with difficult birth and may spread like wildfire, often causing death or loss of fertility. The preventive is to control abortion and use strict sanitary procedures during lambing.
18. Mastitis, or inflammation of the udder, may be due to any one of several types of infection. It may be fatal or lead to partial or complete loss of ability to nurse young. Prevention demands strict sanitary measures, particularly in goat dairies.
19. Prolapsis is a misplacement or eversion of the vagina or uterus, due to severe strain or rough handling during lambing. It is fatal if treatment, which consists largely of careful manipulation, is delayed until general intoxication sets in from stoppage of body functions.
20. Venereal infection of the male or female genital organs in sheep is primarily due to a virus. Antiseptic treatment is generally beneficial if begun early. Control demands thorough sanitary measures.

21. Orchitis, or inflammation of the testicles, caused by injury, excessive service, or infection, may be fatal or lead to impotence. Treatment and control depend on the cause; where a definite infection has been identified, bacterins or other biological products may be useful.

Diseases of the Eye

22. Wool blindness, caused by wool growing close to the eyes, may be prevented by breeding sheep without this characteristic and by suitable trimming.
23. Entropion, an inversion of the eyelid over the eyeball, is treated by surgery. It may be hereditary and hence avoidable by controlled breeding.
24. Foreign bodies may become imbedded in the eye tissues. They should be removed and suitable treatment should be given.
25. Infectious keratitis, or pink eye, which sometimes spreads rapidly in a flock, causes acute inflammation and may end in blindness. It demands isolation and careful treatment of affected animals.

Other Infectious Diseases

26. Arthritis, or inflammation of the joints, probably most common in lambs and rare in goats, is usually caused by infection of the navel stump at birth, or of wounds caused by castration, docking, shearing, or ear-marking. Pus-forming organisms or the swine erysipelas organism are usually involved. Acute cases may be rapidly fatal; others may become chronic. Prevention depends on the use of proper sanitary measures and disinfection.
27. Black disease (infectious necrotic hepatitis) is an acute malady of mature sheep due to infection of the liver by a specific germ which accompanies infestation by liver flukes. Affected animals sometimes die overnight without any sign of illness, and recovery is rare. Prevention depends on the control of flukes.
28. Caseous lymphadenitis is a widespread chronic disease chiefly affecting the lymph glands; it is caused by a bacillus that may enter the body in various ways. There is no

practical treatment. Prevention depends partly on good sanitation.

29. Paratyphoid dysentery, caused by infection with a *Salmonella* organism, is comparatively rare in sheep and can probably be largely prevented by proper care of animals during shipment.

30. Lamb dysentery, or white scours, is a disease of very young animals that may kill 20 to 40 percent of the lamb crop in severe outbreaks. It is essentially filth-borne and is attributed to any one of several micro-organisms. Medicinal treatment is usually useless. Prevention depends on strict sanitation and good management.

31. Johne's disease, or paratuberculosis, is discussed under Diseases of Cattle, and requires the same kind of control measures when it occurs in sheep as when it occurs in cattle.

32. Necrobacillosis is caused by a tissue-killing organism that enters through wounds or very commonly through the lesions produced by other diseases. As a secondary invader, it may greatly complicate the primary malady. Treatment is often unsatisfactory. Strict sanitation is the best preventive.

33. Wound infections, as the author points out, cause enormous losses that could be largely prevented by proper care and disinfection during various operations and in lambing. Many micro-organisms can infect wounds, and some, such as those that cause malignant edema, lockjaw, and blackleg, are very deadly.

Miscellaneous Non-infectious Diseases

34. Goiter, a nutritional disease caused by lack of iodine, is briefly discussed here and in more detail elsewhere in the Yearbook.

35. Urinary calculi (sand, gravel) are, mineral aggregations in the kidneys, ureters, bladder, or urethra. Unless the condition is relieved, it causes death, but treatment is generally not practicable.

36. Stiff lambs (white muscle disease) is a peculiar degeneration of the muscles, usually affecting winter or early spring lambs. The cause is unknown, and there is no successful treatment, but the trouble can be prevented to some extent by good feeding and management.

Internal Parasites of Sheep and Goats

Dikmans and Shorb deal in considerable detail with some 40 internal parasites of sheep and goats, classified as protozoa (minute, one-celled animals), flukes, tapeworms, and roundworms. These parasites attack many parts of the body, including the esophagus, rumen, abomasum, small intestine, cecum, colon, trachea, bronchi, carotid and mesenteric arteries, tear ducts, liver, bile ducts, mesentery, brain and spinal cord, lungs, and voluntary muscles. In general they are a greater menace in the farm areas than in the range areas, partly because of greater crowding in the former, partly because of climatic conditions.

Of the four main groups mentioned, flukes, tapeworms, and some protozoa spend part of their lives in an intermediate host. Most roundworms, on the other hand, do not; they live on the ground during the stages when they are not in the principal host. Only at a certain stage of their development on the ground can roundworm larvae infect sheep and goats.

The symptoms of parasitic infection are usually complicated because more than one species of parasite is present at the same time. In a few experiments it has been possible to bring about "pure" infections with one parasite only, and these have thrown considerable light on symptoms. In general the typical symptoms of worm infestation include unthriftiness, loss of weight, diarrhoea, anemia, potbelly, and bottle jaw.

Two types of protozoa are discussed by these authors.

1. Coccidia, attack the wall of the small intestine. In a resting, or spore, state (oöcysts) they are discharged in the droppings. Probably almost all lambs become infested; light infestations seem to do little harm, but severe ones result in marked symptoms and may be fatal. There is evidence that heavy infestations can be built up in feed lots if feed is handled in such a way that the lambs can continually re-contaminate it. Lowered resistance from various causes, as well as heavy infestations, may have much to do with the severity of the symptoms of coccidiosis.
2. A protozoan (*Globidium gilruthi*) for which there is no common name occurs in the fourth stomach and small intestine of sheep, causing severe symptoms only when the infestation is heavy.

Two kinds of flukes occur in the liver and two in the rumen, or paunch. Eggs of flukes pass out in the droppings and hatch in water. The embryonic flukes then enter snails and develop to a larval stage. Leaving the snails, the larvae, now enclosed in a cyst, attach themselves to vegetation and are swallowed by grazing animals.

The common liver fluke, which infests the liver, bile duct, and gall bladder, is one of the worst parasitic enemies of sheep, severe infestations sometimes causing death in a few days. Common symptoms include loss of condition, anaemic-looking mucous membranes, stiff gait, swellings under the jaw, potbelly. The liver may be greatly damaged. The large American liver fluke, another species, is primarily a parasite of deer, but when it attacks sheep it causes severe symptoms. The rumen flukes, which infest the paunch, have life histories like that of the common liver fluke, but under natural conditions they apparently do not parasitise sheep in the United States.

Several species of tapeworms infest sheep, some as mature worms, some as larvae, a stage in which they are called bladder worms.

Two common adult tapeworms (moniezias) that infest the small intestine pass part of their lives in the bodies of beetle mites, which take up the eggs contained in sheep droppings. Experiments indicate that these tapeworms in themselves do not have such serious effects on lambs as they are usually believed to have. The effects are serious, however, when other parasites are present at the same time.

The adult fringed tapeworm infests the small intestine, bile duct, gall bladder, and sometimes the pancreatic duct. Nothing is known about its life history and little about its effects on sheep.

A bladder worm does not look like an adult tapeworm but like a sac into which the head of the worm is inserted. The sacs may be very large, sometimes several inches long. The adult tapeworms infest dogs and related animals, which void the eggs. Sheep pick up the eggs from contaminated ground.

In sheep the thin-necked bladder worm starts in the liver but eventually attaches itself to certain abdominal membranes; severe infestations make an animal very sick and may be fatal. Another bladder worm, which primarily infests the heart, diaphragm, and various muscles, causes a condition known as sheep measles, which is usually not serious but makes infested meat subject to condemnation in meat-packing plants. The gid bladder worm, sometimes larger than a hen's egg, infests the brain and less often the spinal cord, causing severe nervous disturbances, brain fever, and death. Another bladder worm, the hydatid, usually attacks the liver and lungs but may be found almost anywhere in the body, including the heart and brain. The symptoms depend on the location and size of the parasites.

Except where liver flukes are prevalent, Dikmans and Shorb point out, the roundworms are the most serious parasites of sheep and goats. There are many kinds, infesting different parts of the body.

The most serious of the roundworms in its effects (and therefore the most serious of all sheep parasites) is the twisted stomach worm, which infests the abomasum, or fourth stomach. The eggs of this worm pass out with the droppings, and the infective larvae, which are quite resistant to unfavourable climatic conditions except drought, are taken up by sheep with contaminated feed and water. Symptoms in severe cases include great weakness, anemia, and bottle jaw; sudden death sometimes occurs following a heavy infestation acquired in a short period of time.

A number of smaller worms, called small trichostrongyles, infest the abomasum and small intestine. The larvae of some of these worms are able to survive long periods of drought and resume their development on pastures as soon as moisture becomes available. Essentially, they cause a slow, protracted disease of your animals, characterized by unthriftiness, diarrhoea, and anemia. Death may result from a severe infestation.

The sheep hookworm enters the body by way of the mouth but can also penetrate the skin. It extracts blood from the animal and also secretes a substance that destroys red corpuscles and prevents coagulation, so that prolonged internal hemorrhages may occur at the points where the worms have been attached. Anemia, dropsical swellings, and unthriftiness are common effects of hookworm infestation.

The thread-necked strongyles, which also infest the small intestine, are apparently not of great importance as disease producers except when the infestations are very large.

A number of roundworms infest the cecum, or blind gut, and the colon. The whipworm apparently causes no marked visible symptoms in sheep. The nodular worm, on the other hand, produces nodules, or lumps, throughout the length of the intestine, making them unfit for sausage casings and surgical-suture material, and can cause severe clinical symptoms. The large-mouthed bowel worm, which infests the colon, may produce diarrhoea, slow growth, and cause weakness and emaciation, but usually these symptoms gradually disappear.

Two roundworms–the thread lungworm and the hair lungworm–infest the respiratory tract. They lay their eggs in the lungs. The larvae develop, are coughed up and swallowed, and pass out with the droppings. The larvae of the thread lungworm develop to an infective stage on the ground, are swallowed by grazing sheep, bore through the small intestine, and reach the lungs by way of the lymph stream. The irritation caused by these worms produces a cough, and heavy infestations may result in suffocation, bronchitis, pneumonia, and death. The larvae of the hair lungworm penetrate into and develop in certain species of snails. Infested sheep do not show the marked symptoms that result from infection by the thread lungworm.

Certain small roundworms parasitize the eyes of ruminants, and one has been reported in sheep, causing abnormal sensitiveness to light, profuse watering of the eyes, and perhaps more severe symptoms. A careful examination of the eye will reveal the worms, and they can be removed mechanically.

Roundworms also occur in the circulatory system. The adults produce no known symptoms, but their larvae, or immature stages, are reported to cause an inflammation of the skin.

Medication and preventive measures are both important in controlling the parasites of sheep and goats, these authors point out.

There is no specific medicinal treatment for coccidiosis. Affected animals should be isolated, soiled feed or other material should be burned or otherwise disposed of, and the premises should be cleaned and disinfected. Feed should be so handled as not to become constantly contaminated.

The medicine commonly used to rid sheep of adult flukes is carbon tetrachloride. Occasionally it is toxic, and it should be used with the precautions outlined by the authors. Fluke infestations can be effectively reduced by wiping out the snail host of the parasite and thereby breaking its life cycle. This involves adequate drainage, where practicable, to dry up wet ground, or the treatment of streams, lakes, and swamps in snail-infested areas with copper sulphate.

Roundworms are attacked by medication with any one of several drugs: Phenothiazine, copper sulphate, tetrachlorethylene, or a combination of copper sulphate and nicotine solution. Dikmans and Shorb list the worms for which each of the drugs seems to be effective, and also those for which there is at present no really effective medicinal treatment. (The latter include the lungworms, the gullet worms, and the fringed tapeworm).

The authors recommend that sheep be treated during the winter to prevent pasture contamination in the spring. Other recommendations include frequent rotation of pasture, avoidance of low-lying, wet pastures, and maintaining a good nutritional state. To prevent bladder worm infection, all infected sheep carcasses and parts should be properly disposed of, stray dogs should be eliminated, and dogs on the place should be periodically examined and wormed when necessary.

The last part of the article is devoted to a discussion of the sheep nasal fly, the grub of which is an internal parasite infesting the nasal passages and frontal sinuses. Bacterial infection follows, resulting in the condition known as snotty nose. Repellents placed in the nasal passages are of little or no value in keeping away infestations of the grub. The authors describe several treatments, including injections, that have been reported to give satisfactory results in clearing up infections.

Sheep Scab and Its Control

Fifty years ago, sheep scab was the worst problem our sheepmen faced; many ranchers would not raise sheep because of the prevalence of scab, and England prohibited the importation of live sheep from the United States. Ninety percent of the flocks in some States were infected. Today, thanks to rigid inspection, quarantine, and required dipping, most of the range States in which sheep are important are entirely free of the diseases. It is still a serious problem among farm flocks in areas where auction markets and truck transportation have made eradication difficult, but this problem too is being gradually solved by Federal and State cooperation. Miller advises that every flock owner report the appearance of sheep scab immediately to the nearest veterinarian. State livestock official, or Bureau of Animal Industry representative and that the dipping be done under veterinary or other expert supervision. Only lime-sulphur or nicotine solutions are allowed for official dipping, and the dip must be of a specified strength.

Four kinds of mange mites cause sheep scab. The psoroptic mite, living on the surface of the skin, causes common scab, which covers extensive areas over the body, including the withers, back, sides, and rump. The sarcoptic mites, which are not common in the United States, burrow into the skin, usually attacking the head and face where there is little or no wool. The chorioptic mites live on the surface and usually attack the legs. The demodectic mites live in the hair follicles and glands of the skin, producing pimples or nodules. Miller describes the symptoms of the different kinds of scab, but a definite diagnosis should be based on finding the mites.

Of the four kinds of scab, demodectic is incurable; affected animals can be removed from the flock and treated by carefully opening and disinfecting each nodule, or the animals can be destroyed. Sarcoptic (head) scab is difficult to eradicate but can be cured by soaking the affected parts with warm lime-and-sulphur dip every 5 or 6 days for a month or 6 weeks. Chorioptic (foot) and psoroptic (common) scab are cured by dipping, but during very cold weather a wading tank instead of a dipping vat may be used for foot scab.

Miller goes into considerable detail regarding the method of dipping in lime-and-sulphur or nicotine solution. In particular, there are various precautions that must be carefully observed if the job is to be done satisfactorily and danger or injury to the sheep is to be avoided.

Sheep Ticks

Sheep ticks–which are not true ticks but wingless flies–are, widespread in the United States and attack both sheep and Angora goats. puncturing the skin to suck blood, causing damage to fleeces, and injuring the health of lambs and kids. The ticks do not lay eggs but give birth to larvae enclosed in a membrane that soon becomes a hard puparium and is attached to the wool fibers by a gluelike substance. Ticks spread rapidly in a flock, especially when the sheep are crowded together during cold weather.

Two general types of dips are used to control the parasites, With the first type, consisting of a solution of nicotine, or coal-tar creosote, or cresol, the sheep must be dipped twice; the second dipping is made 24 to 28 days after the first to catch the new crop of ticks hatching out from the pupae not killed by the first dipping. The other type of dip (fused bentonite-sulphur-cube, or arsenic-sulphur-rotenone, or derris, or cube) remains active in the fleece long enough to kill the new ticks emerging from the pupae, so that a second dipping is unnecessary. In their article, Imes and Babcock give general directions for using both types of dips.

Since the pupae can remain alive off the sheep for about 60 days during warm weather, it is important to clean and disinfect quarters that have been occupied by ticky sheep and to keep clean sheep out of infested pastures for about 2 months.

Goat Lice

Lice are the worst external parasites of goats in this country; yet the widespread damage they do every year is unnecessary because they can be easily eradicated. All told, five species of lice infest goats, of which two are bloodsuckers and three have mouth parts fitted only for chewing. All reproduce by means of eggs, which are attached to the hair fibers. Heavily infested animals lose weight and become unthrifty, and in the case of Angora goats both the quality and the quantity of mohair are greatly reduced. The lice spread rapidly in a herd.

The only certain method of eradication is to dip the entire herd, using a solution of wettable sulphur (preferably mixed with cube or derris powder) or an arsenical or coal-tar-creosote dip. For a small number of animals, a large washtub or a small galvanized iron tank will suffice; for a large number it is necessary to have a regular dipping vat. The best time to dip Angora goats is a mouth to 6 weeks after they are sheared; provided this is before the arrival of cold weather; other breeds may be dipped at any time when the weather is favourable. The authors give general directions for dipping, including the precautions that should be observed.

If a heavy infestation makes treatment of a few animals necessary during the winter, they may be hand-dusted, or sprayed, with a combination of sulphur and derris or cube. Although this will not eradicate the lice, it will greatly lessen their numbers.

Pregnancy Disease of Sheep

"The death of one or more ewes just before lambing time is sufficient to justify suspicion of pregnancy disease," says Shahan. The first signs of the disease, which strikes for the most part during the last month of pregnancy, usually include grinding of the teeth, dullness, weakness, frequent urination, trembling when exercised; the final stage is complete collapse, followed by death in 90 percent of the cases. Affected ewes are almost invariably those carrying more than one fetus, and they are usually animals between 3 and 6 years of age.

The specific cause of pregnancy disease is not known, but it is attributed to disturbances in metabolism; and this is supported by the fact that the disease is accompanied by an increase in certain complex acids (ketones) in the blood and urine and a decrease in blood sugar. (Laboratory analysis may detect these changes even before visible symptoms appear.) Prevention consists in (1) giving the ewes a good ration during the strain of pregnancy, with its greatly increased demands on the body, and (2) seeing to it that they get regular, moderate exercise during this period. Shahan, gives suggestions for the kind of ration that should be used to avoid both undernourishment and overfeeding.

Lunger Disease of Sheep

Lunger Disease, found mostly among range sheep in the Northwest, is chronic progressive pneumonia, incurable at present and generally considered to be fatal in all cases. The symptoms include laboured and rapid breathing, pumping (flank breathing), dilated nostrils, sometimes coughing and a nasal discharge, and finally great weakness and emaciation before death. Investigators in the United States and in South Africa, where a similar disease occurs, have attributed it to various micro-organisms, but the cause has not even definitely determined as yet. Possibly certain environmental conditions make the animals especially susceptible. In the absence of any known method of prevention or treatment, Creech advises separating affected sheep from the healthy ones as a precaution and, if possible, moving the flock to a new environment.

Chapter 1

FOOT ROT OF SHEEP

M.S. Shahan[1]

[1] *M.S. Shahan is Veterinarian, Pathological Division, Bureau of Animal Industry.*

Foot Rot, due to infection in the hoofs of sheep and goats, is a rather widespread and sometimes serious disease that cripples the animals and causes great suffering. It yields well to combined surgical and medicinal treatment, and much can be done to prevent it.

Foot Rot is a specific infectious disease that periodically becomes a major hazard to sheep raising and sheep feeding over wide areas in the United States. It has also been reported from many other countries where sheep husbandry is important. In this country the disease is especially troublesome in flocks confined in crowded corrals or pastures, but it occasionally affects range sheep as well, especially during exceptionally wet seasons. Goats are sometimes affected by a similar, if not identical, disease.

Symptoms

Usually the first indication of the disease to be observed is lameness in some of the sheep in the flock or band, but before this becomes marked there is usually reddening and swelling of the skin just above the hoof, between the toes, or at the bulb of the heel. More or less oozing of watery fluid from the inflamed tissues follows, and if the disease is not stopped the sole and walls of the affected foot are undermined by the infectious process. Death of the tissues results in the accumulation of a grayish-yellow, cheesy exudate, or discharge, followed by separation of the hoof from the underlying sensitive tissues. A characteristic foul odour is invariably present.

If the disease is allowed to progress, lameness becomes more and more pronounced. One foot or all may be involved. When both forefeet are affected, the pain may be so intense that the animal kneels to feed. If all four feet are severely affected, the animal may refuse to stand. The infection penetrates deeper and deeper into the tissues until not only the ligaments and tendons but even the bones and joints may be involved. In warm weather the feet may become infested with maggots.

Some severely affected sheep may die, but even the worst cases sometimes gradually improve after several weeks, seeming to recover even without treatment. But within the long, misshapen, and extremely hard hoofs or beneath the fungoid masses that may develop between the toes, the infection often remains, to break out again in the flock. The condition tends to improve when sheep are on dry, well-drained land, but unless it is eliminated by treatment, the disease is likely to persist in affected flocks for months or even years.

Cause

Foot rot can be readily transmitted to healthy sheep by inoculating them with exudate from the feet of affected animals. Because the feet of sheep are constantly exposed to the myriads of germs present in soil, manure, and water, bacteriological studies of the disease are difficult. In foot rot, pus-forming bacteria, colon bacilli, spirochetes, and other micro-organisms are frequently present.

The micro-organism known as *Actinomyces necrophorus*, which destroys the tissues it affects, is frequently found in cases of foot rot (*6, 7*)[2], and it is considered by some the essential cause of the disease. An organism known as *Treponema podovis*, or *Spirochaeta penortha*, and by other names is commonly present (*1, 3, 4, 5*). A germ which is known tentatively as *Fusiformis nodosus* has lately been assigned the causative role in the disease (*2*) with a suggestion that other

---

[2] Italic numbers in parentheses refer to Literature Cited.

organisms, particularly spirochetes and the tissue-destroying bacillus mentioned, probably act as accessories or secondary factors. The apparent confusion among qualified investigators as to the exact cause of the disease is probably largely due to the indiscriminate use of the term "foot rot" for almost any abnormal condition of the feet associated with lameness.

Treatment

Although the cause of the disease may not yet be wholly agreed upon by veterinary investigators, fortunately there are definite principles of treatment which, if followed, are very successful. As with most other animal diseases, it is preferable that treatment and preventive measures be applied by a veterinarian, or at least under the direction and supervision of a veterinarian.

Of primary importance is the immediate examination at the first signs of foot rot of all sheep in the band or flock and the segregation of all animals showing any symptoms. At this time any excessive or abnormal growth of hoof should be pared away with a sharp knife or pruning shears. Hoof nippers may be required in some cases. The object should be not only to restore the normal proportions and contour of the hoof but also to discover so far as possible any evidence of the foot rot infection.

In a typical, well-established case the affected animal will usually be found to have deep-seated infections beneath the sole or the hoof wall. Proper treatment demands the removal of such parts of the hoof as are undermined by the typical grayish, dead tissue characteristic of the disease (Fig. 1). Trimming sometimes assumes the proportions of a major surgical operation. The tendency of the average untrained or inexperienced person is to trim either too little or too much of the horny hoof. If too little is taken away, the depths of the infected tissue cannot be reached by the antiseptic which is subsequently applied. Too drastic trimming and paring, on the other hand, needlessly injure normal tissues and thus still further delay healing.

After the feet have been trimmed, a suitable antiseptic should be applied. If a good job of trimming has been done, nearly any efficient antiseptic agent may suffice to curb the infection. If only a few animals are to be treated, their feet may be immersed in a bucket or other receptacle containing the antiseptic, or the antiseptic may

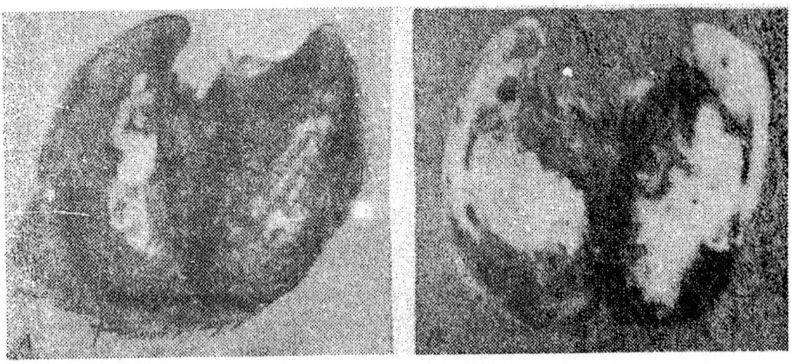

Fig. 1: The foot of a sheep affected with foot rot: *A*: Before trimming; *B*: after trimming. (Courtesy of the Montana Agricultural Experiment Station).

be applied by hand. The choice of method, as well as the selection of an antiseptic, depends on the severity and extent of the disease and the facilities available for handling the sheep. *Severely caustic chemicals should never be used by inexperienced persons.*

When large numbers of sheep are to be treated, a trough of wood or other convenient material is usually constructed for use as a foot bath in applying the antiseptic. For most sheep an inside width of about 12 inches and a depth of 6 to 8 inches is adequate. The length of the trough depends on the number of sheep. A 10-foot trough is long enough for a small flock, but one considerably longer is preferable if several hundred sheep are to be treated. The trough may be placed along a corral fence or in a gateway. Converging wing panels or hurdles, either permanent or movable, are usually provided at the entrance to facilitate handling the sheep. Outwardly sloping panels are usually placed at the sides of the trough in a chutelike arrangement. The length of time each sheep should stand in the loot bath depends on the nature and strength of the antiseptic used and the extent of the disease. These matters are best judged by the attending veterinarian. Ordinarily no sheep is kept in the trough for less than 1 minute, and longer than 5 minutes is rarely necessary or advisable. In any event, the animals should be closely watched to insure immersion of the feet and to prevent them from lying down in the trough.

The substance most widely used in treating foot rot is a solution of copper sulphate, or so-called bluestone. The chemical, preferably in powdered form, is dissolved in warm or hot water in 10- to 30-percent solutions (about 4/5 to 2½ pounds per gallon), prepared preferably in enameled or earthenware vessels. When weak solutions are used, the sheep should ordinarily be held longer in the foot bath. The strongest solution may be effective in one application, while two or more treatments at 2- to 4-day intervals may be required if less concentrated solutions are used.

Some cases respond well to treatment with 2- to 10-percent dilutions of formaldehyde solution (U.S.P). *This, as well as copper sulphate, is very irritating to human beings, as well as to the animals, and it should be handled with care.* Other drugs are applicable in individual cases, depending on the extent of the disease and the facilities available for handling the animals to be treated. The longer treatment is delayed, the greater will be the likelihood of serious loss.

In practice, some use another trough, containing water only, placed at the front end of that containing the antiseptic. This water bath washes dirt from the sheep's feet before they enter the medicinal bath. If the disease is advanced and the feet are extremely sensitive after treatment, they may well be protected by clean, soft dressings and the application of some such substance as oil of pine tar.

Prevention

As with other infectious diseases, prevention is much more effective than is treatment after the disease has developed. Because infected sheep are considered the greatest source of infection, any sheep to be added to a flock from outside sources should first be held in quarantine for at least a month. If no indications of foot rot appear by the end of the quarantine period, usually the new animals may safely be added to the flock. Sheep should preferably be procured from a source known to have been free of foot rot for at least 6 months previously. Sheep treated for the disease should not be returned to the flock until it is certain that they are normal. In some cases the most economical procedure may be to sell all affected sheep for slaughter under inspection, thus eliminating the expense of treatment and the hazard of their presence to the healthy sheep.

Barns, sheds, troughs, and corrals that have been used by infected sheep should be thoroughly cleaned and disinfected. All accumulations of litter and manure should be removed and preferably burned. Infective foot trimmings and dressings also should be disposed of by burning. Muddy corrals and pastures should be drained, if practicable. In severely affected flocks it may be advisable to move all the apparently normal sheep to fresh ground. It is not known exactly how long land used by sheep affected with foot rot remains infectious. If the soil is light and well-drained, the rainfall limited, and the weather hot with an abundance of sunshine, the infection will probably not survive for more than 2 weeks. Under such conditions corrals may ordinarily be considered safe from the standpoint of foot rot if sheep are excluded for a month. On the other hand, if the soil is heavy and poorly drained and there is much rainfall and a scarcity of sunshine, a considerably longer time may be necessary before sheep can be safely returned. In northern latitudes, infected pastures are generally considered safe if sheep are withheld for 4 months during the usual cold winter season.

If different attendants cannot be provided for the healthy sheep and for those being treated for foot rot, the normal sheep should be cared for first and the others last. After handling affected sheep, attendants should cleanse themselves and disinfect all instruments used.

As an added measure of prevention, the apparently healthy portion of the band is sometimes subjected to the antiseptic foot bath described. When this is done, old solutions that have been used by infected sheep should not be used for the healthy sheep.

Conditions Confused with Foot Rot

Animals compelled to travel long distances over rough, hard, gravelly, or rocky roads or trails, or those pastured on exceptionally dry, sparse pastures, frequently develop foot soreness that may be confused with foot rot. Continuously stabled animals or those pastured on low-lying, swampy lands are apt to develop grotesquely shaped, overgrown hoofs, which should be trimmed periodically to prevent lameness. Sheep pastured on muddy ground often collect caked and dried soil between the toes, with resulting injury to the tissues, which may become more or less severely infected. Sheep on stubblefields not infrequently suffer from local injuries that are likewise avenues for the entrance of nonspecific infections. Injuries due to penetrating wounds usually occur only in one or a few animals at a time and are readily identified. The treatment of all such animals is made easier and more effective if they are confined or isolated, just as they would be if foot rot were present.

Literature Cited

(1) BEVERIDGE, W.I.B. (1936). A STUDY OF SPIROCHAETA PENORTHA (N. SP.) ISOLATED FROM FOOT-ROT IN SHEEP. Austral. Jour. Expt. Biol. and Med. Sci. 14: [307]-318, illus.

(2) _____(1941). FOOT-ROT IN SHEEP: A TRANSMISSIBLE DISEASE DUE TO INFECTION WITH FUSIFORMIS NODOSUS (N. SP.). Austral. Council Sci. and Indus. Res. Bul. 140, 56 pp., illus. [Processed].

(3) BLAIZOT, LUDORIC, and BLAIZOT, PIERRE (1928). TREPONEMA PODOVIS N. SP., AGENT PATHOGENE DU PIETIN DES MOUTONS. [Paris] Acad. des Sci. Compt. Rend. 187: 911-912.

(4) HOWARTH, J.A. (1930). FOOT ROT IN SHEEP. Vet. Med. 25: 186-188, illus.

(5) _____(1930). THE PATHOGENIC SIGNIFICANCE OF SPIROCHETES IN SOME WELL-KNOWN PATHOLOGICAL CONDITIONS OF DOMESTIC ANIMALS. Amer. Vet. Med. Assoc. Jour. 76: 630-642, illus.

(6) MARSH, HADLEIGH, and TUNNICLIFF, E.A. (1934). EXPERIMENTAL STUDIES OF FOOT-ROT IN SHEEP. Mont. Agr. Expt. Sta. Bul. 285, 29 pp., illus.

(7) MOHLER, JOHN R., and WASHBURN, HENRY J. (1904). FOOT-ROT OF SHEEP: ITS NATURE, CAUSE, AND TREATMENT. U.S. Bur. Anim. Indus. Bul. 63, 39 pp., illus.

Chapter 2

SORE MOUTH OF SHEEP AND GOATS

M.S. Shahan[1]

[1] *M.S. Shahan is Veterinarian, Pathological Division, Bureau of Animal Industry.*

Sore Mouth, a virus disease that attacks young animals especially, is serious partly because it so often lead to complications with other infections. It can be controlled, as this article makes clear, by sanitary measures and the use of preventive vaccination.

Sore Mouth is widely prevalent among lambs in feed lots and is considered by some authorities to be almost always present to some degree wherever lambs are fattened for the market. The disease also occurs in range bands and farm flocks and not uncommonly affects goats, particularly kids. Technically, it is known as contagious ecthyma.

Cause and Symptoms

Sore mouth is a highly contagious disease caused by a specific filtrable virus (*1, 3, 5, 7*)[2], which is capable of remaining infective for months in the dried scabs that develop in the course of the illness.

---

[2] Italic numbers in parentheses refer to Literature Cited.

The affection seldom appears in animals over 1 year old. Lambs shipped to the feed lot frequently develop the disease, usually within a week to 10 days after arrival. Small vesicles appear on the lips, gums, or tongue, which are considerably swollen and somewhat reddened. After a few days the vesicles become pustules. These finally rupture, leaving raw, granulating sores, that bleed easily and are encrusted with thick, grayish-brown scabs (Fig. 1). Within 3 to 4 weeks the scabs drop off, and the lesions heal, leaving no scars.

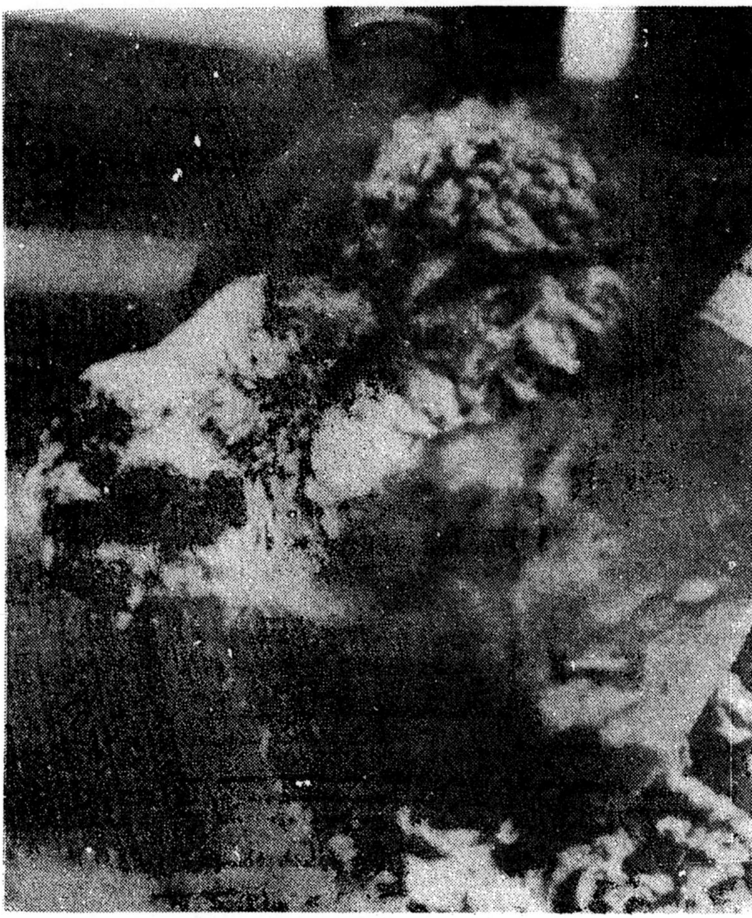

Fig. 1: A sheep affected with sore mouth. (Courtesy of the Colorado Agricultural Experiment Station).

This description applies to the typical uncomplicated case. The chief trouble caused by such an infection is the extreme soreness of the affected parts. Lambs or kids nurse reluctantly, and older animals graze with difficulty and even at the trough may eat sparingly. In consequence growth is more or less impaired, and considerable weight may be lost. Death from the disease is rare.

Occasionally bacterial infection; chiefly by *Actinomyces necrophorus*, takes place (*4*). In such instances, areas of dead tissue frequently develop in the stomach and intestines, the liver, or the lungs. The death loss from such so-called secondary infection may reach 50 percent of the animals affected. In some sections of the country, infestations of the lesions, or injuries, of sore mouth with screwworms is a common trouble.

The lesions of contagious ecthyma, with or without complicating bacterial infection, sometimes appear on the udders of nursing ewes and goats, and the resulting soreness may lead to the animals, refusing to permit their young to nurse. Then, either through the accumulation of milk in the udder or bacterial, infection or both, caked udder, mastitis, or "blue bag" may develop. Sometimes the eyelids are involved, and the sight is threatened. Contagious ecthyma has also been reported to produce lesions on the ears, under the tail, on the inside of the thighs, or in other areas where there is little wool or hair.

Prevention

Before the vaccine now used was developed, isolation of affected animals and general sanitation of corrals, barns, sheds, etc., were the only practicable means of controlling sore mouth. These measures are still to be considered effective adjuncts in the prevention and control of the disease, and they may be followed without using vaccine in flocks where the veterinarian considers this procedure advisable.

The vaccine now commercially available was developed at the Texas Agricultural Experiment Station (*1, 2, 7*) between 1932 and 1935. Made from the scabs taken from typical cases, it is similar in nature to smallpox vaccine and is applied to scratches in the skin on the under side of the tail, the inside of the thigh, or elsewhere. Susceptible animals develop takes resembling the lesions of the natural disease, and after recovery they are immune, with relatively few exceptions, for several months to 2 years or longer. Animals that have recovered from the disease itself are similarly immune.

In range areas where the disease is known to prevail, a practical procedure has been to have the lambs or kids vaccinated at the time of marking, that is, when castration, docking, and earmarking are done, though sometimes this may not be wise or convenient for various reasons. It has been found that the disease can be almost entirely prevented in feed-lot sheep if they are vaccinated at least 10 days before being shipped (2, 6). Immunity thus has time to develop before exposure to infection during shipping.

Since the scab that falls away from the site of the vaccination contains the causative virus just as does the scab from a natural case, sheep should not be shipped until after the vaccination wounds have completely healed. Delay until then is believed to result also in a more complete resistance to any infection that might be acquired enroute. Because the virus may be distributed around premises where vaccine has been used, either through accident in handling the vaccine or the falling of the scabs from the vaccinated animals, vaccine should never be used except in areas or on premises where the disease has been diagnosed by a veterinarian.

The disease spreads so rapidly in feed lots, and occasionally on the range or farm, that vaccination after it appears is rarely practical. There may be some benefit from vaccination, however, if it is done promptly before many of the animals have developed symptoms.

Treatment

As indicated in the discussion of symptoms, treatment, except for isolation of the affected animals in clean, roomy quarters, is usually unnecessary. The disease runs its course, and medicinal aid is seldom required and rarely practical. The chief considerations are the prevention of screwworm infestations and secondary infections. If such complications arise, vigorous treatment with selected larvicides and antiseptics is indicated. The foci of bacterial invasion are usually beyond the reach of any known medicinal agent, but the extensive development of such complications can be largely avoided by local antiseptic treatment. If screwworms infest the lesions, they should be promptly removed.

Literature Cited

(1) BOUGHTON, I.B., and HARDY, W.T. (1934). CONTAGIOUS ECTHYMA (SORE MOUTH) OF SHEEP AND GOATS. Amer. Vet. Med. Assoc. Jour. 85: 150-178, illus.

(2) _____and HARDY, W.T. (1935). IMMUNIZATION OF SHEEP AND GOATS AGAINST SORE MOUTH (CONTAGIOUS ECTHYMA). Tex. Agr. Expt. Sta. Bul. 504, 16 pp., illus.

(3) HOWARTH, J.A. (1929). INFECTIOUS PUSTULAR DERMATITIS OF SHEEP AND GOATS. Amer. Vet. Med. Assoc. Jour. 75: 741-760, illus.

(4) NEWSOM, I.E., and CROSS, FLOYD (1931). SOME COMPLICATIONS OF SORE MOUTH IN LAMBS. Amer. Vet. Med. Assoc. Jour. 78: 539-544.

(5) _____and CROSS, FLOYD (1934). SORE MOUTH IN FEEDER LAMBS DUE TO A FILTRABLE VIRUS. Amer. Vet. Med. Assoc. Jour. 84: 238-247, illus.

(6) _____and THORP, FRANK, JR. (1938). LAMB DISEASES IN COLORADO FEEDLOTS. Colo. Agr. Expt. Sta. Bul. 448, 42 pp., illus.

(7) SCHMIDT, H., and HARDY, W.T. (1932). SOREMOUTH (CONTAGIOUS ECTHYMA) IN SHEEP AND GOATS. Tex. Agr. Expt. Sta. Bul. 457, 22 pp., illus.

Chapter 3

MISCELLANEOUS DISEASES OF SHEEP AND GOATS

M.S. Shahan[1]

[1] *M.S. Shahan is Veterinarian, Pathological Division. Bureau of Animal Industry.*

Here is a discussion of some 36 or more diseases and injuries to which sheep and goats are subject. Many of them, it will be noted, can be largely prevented by good management, proper feeding, strict sanitation, and care in ordinary operations involving surgery. The author emphasizes the need for sound veterinary diagnosis.

Diseases of the Digestive Organs

Bloat, constipation, diarrhoea, and enterotoxemia are included among diseases of the digestive organs. All may be largely prevented or controlled by proper feeding.

Bloat, or the accumulation of gas in the stomach or intestines of sheep and goats from fermentation of their contents, is chiefly the result of feeding green, wet, frosted, or damaged feeds, but it may occur after the eating of any feed in large quantities, particularly one to which the animals are not accustomed. Bloat is an evidence of indigestion and in an acute form it is very troublesome and dangerous. To prevent it, sheep should be given only clean, sound feed in amounts that they can satisfactorily digest. If, through inexperience or accident, the trouble occurs in a flock, all the animals should be immediately removed from access to either feed or water. Kneading the paunch through the abdominal wall in the region of the left flank and slowly driving the affected animal may promote passage of the gas. Elevating the forequarters or placing a gag in the mouth may accomplish the same purpose. If a veterinarian is not available, oil of turpentine (1 to 2 teaspoonfuls) or aromatic spirits of ammonia (½ to 1 teaspoonful) in a half pint of water or milk may be given as a drench. A laxative is generally desirable. When death threatens from extreme distention, an opening into the paunch may be made to permit the escape of the gas. This is usually done by the veterinarian with a special instrument known as a trocar and cannula. In an emergency, the operation may be performed by an untrained person, but, whenever possible, instructions should be obtained from a veterinarian before resorting to this. After recovery from acute bloat, the animal should be allowed free access to water but be given only laxative feeds in small amounts for several days.

Constipation, or impaction of feed in the paunch or the other stomachs, may develop as a result of feeding coarse, dry, or indigestible feed or from overfeeding more healthful materials. The remedy is to remove the accumulated feed by means of drugs that stimulate the muscles of the digestive tract, kneading the flanks, introducing water into; the stomach through a stomach tube, or, if necessary, by drenching or the administration of appropriate laxatives.

Diarrhoea, or watery feces, may be caused by internal parasites such as coccidia or worms, infection by bacteria such as *Salmonella aertrycke* or *Mycobacterium paratuberculosis*, the feeding of green succulent feeds, or excessive consumption of any feed. Prevention and cure depend upon the nature of the underlying cause. Lamb dysentery, paratyphoid dysentery, and Johne's disease are distinctly different from simple diarrhoea and are discussed elsewhere in this article.

Enterotoxemia, intoxication or poisoning of intestinal origin, is probably the most frequent cause of losses of lambs in western feed lots. It differs from the Australian disease of the same name (*1*)[2], though the two are similar in some respects. Feed lot enterotoxemia

---

[2] Italic numbers in parentheses refer to Literature Cited.

results from the overeating of grains or other concentrates. The immediate cause may be the toxin formed in the intestines by the widely distributed germ *Clostridium perfringens* (*Cl. welchii*) (*8*). A similar condition, known as pulpy kidney disease or milk colic, sometimes develops in sucking or weanling lambs pastured on a lush growth of rich forage (*2, 13*).

The prevention of enterotoxemia is essentially a matter of management. A sufficient interval shouid be allowed after placing lambs in the feed lot to permit their digestive organs to become accustomed to the new, rich feed. Different lots of lambs vary widely in their ability to consume feed; what one group will thrive on may be fatal to another. Hence, judgment, skin, and watchfulness are necessary in fattening operations. The ration should be graduated according to the size and condition of the animals being fed, beginning at first with feed consisting chiefly of hay or other roughage, with only a small amount of concentrates, the latter being gradually increased as the animals adapt themselves to the regime. The sheep should be graded according to size and condition, being penned for feeding in as nearly uniform lots as possible.

Once the animals reach the stage of full feed, they should be closely watched. At this time, any disease in the lot will tend to cut down feed consumption by the sick lambs, leaving excessive amounts for the healthy individuals unless the ration is cut in proportion to the number of animals actually on feed. In flocks that develop milk colic on pasture, it is believed to be good practice to reduce the feed of the ewes and lambs by penning them at night and for a part of the day in a dry, clean lot without feed.

Sluggishness, reluctance to eat, and diarrhoea are signs that lambs are going off feed. If the amount of grain is not reduced, considerable losses from death may follow. The animals may be found dead in the pens, a few or many each day, with or without having shown marked signs of abnormality. Sick sheep may be seen with the head elevated, staggering about the pen, running blindly into fences, or in convulsions. Constipation, which may appear early, is usually followed by diarrhoea. At post mortem examination, large hemorrhages may be found in the abdominal cavity, along the intestines, in the diaphragm, or in the belly wall. The inside of the fourth stomach may be reddened. The kidneys and liver may be very friable, or easily torn. In animals that die after a brief illness, few significant abnormalities may be found.

Once lambs have been upset by overfeeding, great difficulty is usually experienced in getting them back into thrifty fattening condition.

While treatment of enterotoxemia is seldom successful and generally uneconomical, the veterinarian should be called to establish the diagnosis and for help in handling the flock in order that further losses may be avoided.

Diseases of the Respiratory System

Respiratory diseases are relatively unimportant in sheep except in connection with shipping, as a result of which hemorrhagic septicemia, or so-called shipping fever, sometimes appears. This is an infectious disease attributed at least in part to the germ *Pasteurella oviseptica*, which is a normal inhabitant of the respiratory passages and usually causes disease only under conditions adverse to the animal's resistance. Such conditions occur when sheep, especially lambs, are taken from grass pastures, shipped crowded together, and subjected to prolonged hunger and perhaps cold, frequently arriving at their destination weak and exhausted. They may be driven considerable distances, becoming overheated, and the feed they are given is usually strange. Young shed-dropped or farm lambs sometimes develop a form of pneumonia much like that of shipping fever.

In feed-lot lambs, shipping fever appears usually within the first few days of the feeding period. As many as half the animals in a shipment may become sick, and the death loss may be 10 percent or more in severe outbreaks (7).

Fever, depression, rapid breathing, sneezing, coughing, and discharge from the eyes and nose are common symptoms. In acute cases, death may result within 24 hours after the illness first appears, and there may be little of diagnostic significance at post mortem examination except perhaps numerous small to large hemorrhages under the skin or within the chest. Chronic cases usually develop into pneumonia, lasting from a few days to several weeks. If death does not intervene, there is a long period of convalescence. Diagnosis of either type of the disease usually depends upon bacteriological examinations.

Improved shipping conditions, including regular rest, feeding, and watering, and protection from severe weather and overcrowding tend to lessen the likelihood of hemorrhagic septicemia in sheep. The disease occurs irregularly, however, from season to season and year to year, and it may develop no matter how well the animals are handled.

Animals may be somewhat protected against the disease by vaccination with hemorrhagic septicemia bacterin, preferably administered some time before they are to be shipped. During years when the disease is prevalent, anti-hemorrhagic-septicemia serum may be given as a preventive. This has a quicker but less prolonged prophylactic effect than bacterin. The decision as to which if any biological product is to be used in each case should be left to the veterinarian familiar with all the circumstances.

Treatment of the disease is generally uneconomical, though serum may be used in selected cases with good results. Prompt isolation and good nursing of affected animals are advantageous.

Exposure of sheep to cold after shearing or dipping may cause pneumonia. Other forms of pneumonia occur as a result of invasion of the lungs by various parasites or bacteria.

Nasal catarrh, or snuffles, is a common condition in sheep, especially those ranging on dry, sparsely vegetated land or travelling dusty trails. The ailment is generally negligible unless it becomes marked, as in pneumonia, severe cases of grub in the head, or specific local infection. Control and treatment under these conditions depend upon the nature of the cause.

Diseases of the Nervous System

Listerellosis (listeriosis), rabies, meningitis, enterotoxemia, paralysis, and gid infection are included among diseases of the nervous system.

Listerellosis, or circling disease, in sheep consists essentially of an inflammation of the brain caused by the germ known as *Listerella monocytogenes*, or *Listeria*. The symptoms of the malady include nervous disorders, inflammation of the eye, and occasionally abortion. Dullness, fever, and strange, awkward movements, such as staggering, pushing the head into fences, and walking in circles, are observed. Paralysis, finally ending in death, follows in most cases.

It is not known how the disease is spread, and there are no proved means of prevention or treatment. Diagnosis depends upon laboratory examinations, since autopsy does not reveal characteristic changes in the body.

Rabies, which may affect any species of mammal. It is referred to here to emphasize that when a nervous disease appears in goats or sheep, the possibility that rabies is the cause should be considered by the veterinarian. Small ruminants with rabies behave much like any other animal affected with the disease, and the symptoms commonly include those seen in other nervous diseases. Licking or gnawing at the site of the bite, stamping of the feet, and bleating are frequently observed. Some animals become belligerent before the final paralysis that ends in death. The prevention of rabies in sheep or goats is essentially the same as in the case of other animals.

Meningitis consists of an inflammation of the meninges, or membranes, which cover the brain within the cranial cavity. It generally accompanies encephalitis, or inflammation of the brain, to a greater or less extent, regardless of the cause of the latter. It is not a specific disease like cerebrospinal meningitis of man but may be caused by any of several micro-organisms. Pus-forming *Staphylococcus*, *Streptococcus*, and other organisms are responsible in some cases. These organisms frequently gain entrance to the body at the time of docking and castration or through the navel at birth and may become localized anywhere in the body. When they become established in the brain or spinal cord, symptoms of nervous disorder, including paralysis, may occur. Such cases are relatively infrequent and may be prevented almost entirely by proper technique in handling the animals during the operations mentioned. Determination of the exact cause of meningitis requires bacteriological study. Treatment is seldom practical.

Paralysis, or loss of the ability to move a part of the body, particularly the legs, rarely occurs except in the course of the diseases mentioned, although it is a common symptom of pregnancy disease and milk fever. Paralysis is sometimes attributed, however, to a toxin or other substance in certain ticks that feed upon sheep. Removal of the ticks usually leads to prompt recovery, as is also true in some cases of tularemia, or rabbit fever, which may be conveyed to sheep by infected ticks. Severe blows, falls, or other injuries sometimes cause fracture or dislocation of the vertebrae, leading to paralysis.

Diseases of the Skin

The commonest cause of abnormalities of the skin of sheep is scabies, or scab. Other conditions that may affect the skin directly or indirectly include purulent dermatitis, ringworm, pox, contagious, ecthyma, maggot infestation, filarial dermatosis, and actinobacillosis..

Purulent dermatitis, as here considered, consists in the invasion of the skin and underlying tissues by pus-forming micro-organisms. The organisms may be introduced by penetrating awns and other parts of grasses and other plants, such as foxtail, needlegrass, wild oats, and alfilaria, or through shearing cuts and other wounds. In severely affected animals, the abscesses formed as a result of the bacterial infection may occur deep in the underlying muscles or even in the abdominal cavity and may lead to pyemia, a form of general poisoning. Prevention consists in avoiding, or limiting as far as possible, objects on the pasture or in feed which may collect in the wool and are capable of penetrating the skin. Shear cuts and other wounds should be treated immediately with tincture of iodine or some other suitable antiseptic.

Ringworm is relatively rare in sheep. It may be due to various species of fungi that require laboratory study for identification. The disease should be distinguished from so-called lumpy wool due to *Actinomyces dermatonomous* (3), a fungus-like organism that produces lumpy wool, as the name indicates, but little or no abnormality of the skin except as a secondary manifestation.

Sheep pox is caused by a filtrable virus resembling but not identical with that which causes smallpox in man.

Sheep pox is characterized by the formation of dark-red papules, which turn into blister-like formations, or vesicles, chiefly on the bare or thinly wooled parts of the body. The vesicles break and become infected with pus-forming germs, which frequently cause death through septic infection. Fortunately, the disease has not become established in the United States.

Actinobacillosis is an infectious disease caused by the germ *Actinobacillus lignieresi*. As it has been observed in sheep, the infection enters the body through the punctures made by the awns or other parts of certain plants, such as needlegrass and prickly-pear. Small pockets of pus form in the tissues beneath the skin, sometimes discharging their contents onto the skin and matting the wool in the regions affected, and sometimes leading to generalized lesions in the internal organs.

Diseases of the skin usually cause more or less itching, manifested by scratching or biting of the affected part. Attending this, there are more or less loss of wool and varying degrees of inflammation of the skin. The exact determination of the cause of the trouble usually requires the services of a veterinarian, who should be consulted as soon as the trouble is first noticed. It can then be determined whether the disease is contagious, and if so, its spread can be limited or entirely prevented.

Diseases Connected with Reproduction

Abortion, the pregnancy toxemias, metritis, mastitis, prolapse of the genital organs, venereal infection, and orchitis are among the diseases connected with reproduction.

Abortion signifies the expulsion from the womb of either living or dead young before the normal time of birth. Damaged feeds, especially those that are moldy, are sometimes held responsible for abortion, and some cases are attributable to generalized infection, toxemia, injury, or undernourishment. Infectious abortion of sheep, unlike that of cattle, is rarely attributable to germs of the *Brucella* genus, being most often caused by *Vibrio fetus, Salmonella, Pasteurella, Listerella,* or coliform organisms which infect the fetus and the fetal membranes. Goats, on the other hand, may suffer from infection with any of these organisms, including *Brucella.* With or without abortion, brucellosis in goats is more dangerous for man than brucellosis in any other animal species.

The interval between infection and abortion varies somewhat with the type of germ causing the trouble and may differ in individual outbreaks. Abortion early in the development of the fetus invariably means a dead lamb or kid. When it occurs later, near the normal time of birth, living young may be born, but they are usually so weak that they live only a few days.

Symptoms indicative of impending abortion may or may not be observed. The disease may develop slowly during the gestation period, finally resulting in depression and loss of appetite just before abortion takes place. There may be a rusty-coloured discharge from the vulva, but usually there are no other symptoms. After abortion, an abnormally bloody discharge sometimes persists for a variable period. There may be serious losses due to septicemia, but generally the females return to apparent good health after a few days. The infection, depending on the type, often remains in the uterus, however, either preventing conception at the next breeding period or jeopardizing subsequent pregnancy.

No treatment is effective in preventing abortion once the infection has become established, but much may be done to prevent the spread of the disease within the band. Animals infected with *Brucella*, and sometimes the other types of organisms responsible for abortion, may be identified by means of agglutination tests. Animals so discovered should be so handled as to prevent exposure of other animals on the premises. This means isolation pending recovery or slaughter. Females showing symptoms of impending abortion and those that have aborted should be immediately isolated from the rest of the flock. The aborted fetus, membranes, and contaminated bedding should be completely burned. The quarters used by aborting animals should afterward be thoroughly cleaned and disinfected. Proper handling of the infected animals, including douching of the genital tract when this is advised by the veterinarian, may decrease the duration of infectivity. Those that have aborted should not be bred until no evidence of active infection remains. Many outbreaks of abortion in ewes caused by *Vibrio fetus* have been definitely associated with stagnant or filthy drinking water, through which the infection has been presumed to spread. Feed free from spoilage, as well as clean running water, should be supplied if possible.

Pregnancy toxemia includes two diseases, pregnancy disease and milk fever, which so closely resemble each other in their symptoms as to appear identical in many cases. Pregnancy disease, occurs prior to lambing. Milk fever may occur just before, just after, or as long as 6 weeks after lambing. Milk fever, also called parturient paresis, occurs much more rarely than pregnancy disease. The symptoms of milk fever in ewes resemble those in cows.

Metritis is defined as inflammation of the uterus. Caused by various types of infection, it accompanies and follows abortion or may develop after dystocia, or difficult parturition. Once it appears in a flock of lambing ewes, it may spread like wildfire unless great care is taken.

The symptoms include a brownish or blood-tinged, sometimes foul-smelling, discharge from the vulva. Depending on the severity of the infectious inflammation, there are varying degrees of fever and depression. The appetite is poor or is lost altogether. The back is often arched, and straining sometimes occurs. Death may follow from severe general intoxication, or septicemia. Less severe cases recover after a time, but fertility may be lost.

To prevent metritis, abortion should be controlled and lambing should be carried out under hygienic conditions. The sheds or barns for lambing are best used for this purpose only and should be thoroughly cleaned and disinfected after the conclusion of operations each season and left unoccupied thereafter. In mild weather, lambing on the range or in the pasture may be preferable to lambing indoors. Attendants of ewes with lamb, especially those assisting at lambing, should keep their persons and clothing meticulously clean.

Treatment, except for nursing, should be left to the veterinarian, as douching of the genital tract with medicinal agents is not without danger. General medication also should be given only by the veterinarian.

Mastitis, mammitis, or garget, signifying an inflammation of the udder, may be caused by one or more of several types of organisms (*Staphylococcus, Streptococcus, Pasteurella*-like, and colon-type organisms). The disease may occur during the lambing season or on the range when the lambs are 3 to 4 months old. It usually develops rapidly and is accompanied by fever, loss of appetite, systemic disturbances, and reddening, swelling, and tenderness of the udder. The milk secretion becomes thick, yellowish, and flaky and is sometimes stained with blood. Abscesses may form in the gland, or gangrene ("blue bag") may develop. Many severely affected animals die, especially if neglected. In those that recover, one or both sides of the udder often fail to function thereafter. When the disease occurs early in the nursing period, lambs whose mothers are affected become undernourished and are likely to die unless given special attention.

Field observations indicate that, like metritis and arthritis, the disease is promoted by insanitary conditions in sheds, corrals, or bed grounds. Older lambs may injure the udder by butting when nursing, making it more susceptible to infection. It is advisable to remove the affected ewes from the flock and hand-feed the lambs or place them with a foster mother. Sheds and corrals should be thoroughly cleaned and disinfected. On the range, bed grounds should be frequently changed. When the type of infection is definitely determined bacteriologically, bacterins or toxoids may aid in prevention.

In the early stages of the disease, the sick ewe may be given a saline cathartic (Epsom or Glauber's salts). The udder may be generally milked out several times a day by hand, and it may be bathed 3 or 4 times a day with a very warm solution of Epsom salts (½ pound in 1 quart of water) applied with cotton or cloths. Internal medication may be prescribed by the veterinarian. Drainage of abscesses or amputation of the udder may become necessary.

Mastitis in milk goats is somewhat different from the disease in ranch or range goats or sheep. Because of the relatively close confinement and the contact between animals, the disease may spread rapidly through the milking herd. Isolation of affected animals, strict hygiene in milking operations, and the other general principles of prevention and treatment of the disease in cattle are usually applicable.

Prolapse of the genital organs (eversion of the vagina or uterus) may occur before or after lambing. Excessively fat, closely confined females, those carrying twins or triplets, or those that are thin and undernourished are more likely to evert the uterus or vagina, usually the latter, than those in a normal, thrifty condition. Ewes or does that have had a difficult or delayed parturition or have been roughly treated in attempts to assist in delivery of young are prone to the condition.

The organs protrude from the vulva as a reddened, shining mass. If the condition is neglected, severe swelling, injury, and infection of the misplaced tissues inevitably develop. In such cases the condition is sooner or later complicated by retention of urine and feces and general intoxication. Delay in treatment until this stage is reached invariably results in the death of the animal.

The remedy is to replace the organs as soon as possible after their eversion is discovered. This usually requires the skin of a veterinarian. If one is not available, the parts may be gently bathed with warm physiological salt solution (a heaping teaspoonful of table salt to a quart of boiled water) and then sprinkled with cold boiled water or ordinary granulated sugar, either of which tends to shrink the congested tissues, thus aiding replacement. Return of the organs is sometimes facilitated by slowly bandaging them from behind forward, thus pressing out the blood and reducing the swelling. Replacement is effected by gentle folding and pressure along the course of the genital passage. Suturing (stitching) of the lips of the vulva or application of a trusslike bandage over the vulva may be required to keep the organs in place.

Venereal infection, as the term implies, is an infectious disease of the genital organs of ewes and rams believed to be spread principally by breeding. The condition, commonly referred to as foul sheath in rams, was for years considered to be a form of necrobacillosis, discussed later in this article, but a filtrable virus has lately been defined as the primary cause (*15*). Ulcers and scabs form on the penis and at the orifice or inside the sheath of the ram and on or about the lips of the vulva in the ewe. Uncomplicated cases recover in several days with few or no serious consequences, but when secondary infection occurs, severe swellings of the affected parts, with pus formation, ulceration, and even gangrene, are not uncommon. In males urination may be greatly restricted, and when this occurs a general septic infection and death may follow.

If begun early in the course of the disease, mild antiseptic treatment is generally beneficial. Neglected or improperly treated animals may be so seriously affected as to warrant destruction. Immediate isolation and treatment of affected animals and thorough cleaning of corrals and disinfection of barns and sheds are advocated for the control of the disease.

Orchitis, or inflammation of the testicle, leads to more orless swelling and tenderness of the organ, with or without systemic disturbance, and sometimes results in impotence or death.

The affected buck walks with a stiff, straddling gait. The testicle becomes acutely inflamed or may be infiltrated with serum or pus. Gangrene may develop.

In large bands of rams the condition arises from injuries caused by fighting, or it may be due to excessive service or infection. Prevention is implemented by sanitation, limiting the ewes for each ram to a reasonable number, regulation of the diet, exercise for rams during the interbreeding season, and finally the separation of fighting animals and their grouping in small lots whenever practicable.

Treatment of orchitis in sheep or goats depends upon the character and extent of the inflammation. Acute injuries may be remedied by confinement, rest, laxative feed, and local applications of a saturated solution of Epsom salts or cold or hot water. If pus forms, it may become advisable to lance the organ, following with antiseptic treatment. In case of gangrene, castration may become necessary. Septicemia resulting from orchitis usually requires general medication.

Bacterins and other biological products may be applicable as preventives in flocks in which the type of infection has been definitely determined.

Diseases of the Eyes

For practical purposes, diseases of the eyes of sheep are of two classes–traumatic (that is, due to injury) and infectious.

Traumatic affections include wool blindness, entropion, and injuries ca used by foreign bodies. The first occurs in sheep with heavily wooled faces. The wool grows over the eyes, obscuring the vision and sometimes injuring the eye tissues. The obvious remedies are to breed sheep without this characteristic or to trim the wool around the eyes periodically.

Entropion consists in an inversion of the eyelid over the eyeball, in consequence of which the eyeball becomes inflamed. This condition is suspected of being hereditary in nature, in which case it could be avoided by careful selection of breeding animals. The remedy is surgery, involving removal of a part of the eyelid, then suturing the organ, or–a more practical procedure–placing a stitch in the lid or tying a fold of the lid with a ligature in such a way as to prevent inversion.

Dust, plant particles, and other foreign substances cause inflammation when they become imbedded in the eye tissues. Healing can be effected only after first removing the offending object.

Infectious keratitis, or pinkeye, is generally considered as an infectious disease that may spread rapidly from one animal to another in a flock or may be carried from one flock to another. There is first a watery discharge from the eye, attended by swelling, reddening, and tenderness of the lids. The conjunctiva (the membrane covering the front surfaces of the eyeball and the inside of the lids) is acutely inflamed, the blood vessels standing out clearly owing to congestion. The discharge later becomes purulent, and the lids are more or less stuck together. The cornea (clear portion of the eye) becomes opaque, appearing smoky or grayish, and at this stage the sheep is blind. This continues for a week or 10 days, when the eye usually clears up if it has been properly treated; otherwise the condition may progress to ulceration of the cornea, which tends to persist and usually results in total blindness. Some animals then die of thirst, hunger, or secondary infection.

To be distinguished from pinkeye is the condition in goats and sheep brought about by a diet low in vitamin A, in which, in addition to unthriftiness and urinary calculi, there may be symptoms of night blindness and sometimes opacity and ulceration of the eye (9).

Animals affected with infectious keratitis should be isolated from the rest of the flock in clean, darkened quarters, from which it is best to exclude flies if possible. Water and laxative, nutritious feed should be readily accessible. A solution or an ointment containing boric acid may be placed in the eyes twice or oftener each day. The same medication may or may not be suitable after removal of foreign bodies or an operation to correct entropion, depending on the nature of the case. In many cases of keratitis confinement and simple medication will suffice to forestall serious complications leading to permanent loss of sight, but it may be preferable to use stronger antiseptics, which should be prescribed by a veterinarian. Since the exact nature of the infectious agent that causes the disease is unknown, there are no specific biological agents for prevention or treatment, but bacterins are sometimes used in attempts to limit the severity of the disease.

Other Infectious Diseases

The following infectious diseases deserve special consideration, in addition to those discussed directly or indirectly in this article.

Arthritis, or inflammation of the joints, sometimes referred to as joint ill, occurs most commonly through infection of the navel stamp at birth, or through wounds caused by castration, docking, shearing, or earmarking. According to available information, the disease is not common in goats. In lambs, streptococci, other pus-forming organisms, and *Erysipelothrix rhusiopathiae* (the cause of swine erysipelas), are the organisms usually involved.

The symptoms depend on the type of infection present, occurring within a week after birth or the operation or several weeks later. The joints, particularly the knee, hock, elbow, and stifle, are more or less swollen and painful. There may be mild to extreme lameness. Fever, with or without the formation of pus in the joints and abscesses in the internal organs, is a fairly regular symptom. Acutely affected lambs may die after a brief illness. In such cases loss of appetite, diarrhoea, and progressive weakness are a part of the clinical picture. Most cases due to *Erysipelothrix rhusiopathiae* tend to become chronic. Recovery from the acute lameness is common, but in such instances more or less damage to the joints and general unthriftiness usually remain.

No treatment can be generally recommended, prevention being the mainstay in combating the disease. Three practices should be assiduously followed, especially on premises long used for sheep or other livestock:

(1) Maintenance of sanitary conditions for lambing,

(2) Disinfection of the navel as soon as possible after birth, and

(3) Avoiding unclean instruments or insanitary methods in castration, docking, and earmarking, afterward turning the lambs out into fresh pasture whenever feasible.

An effective method of preventing infection through the navel is to hold a small, wide-mouthed bottle containing tincture of iodine over the stump of the cord, then turn the lamb over on its back with the bottle held in place, and allow the bottle to remain for a minute or two before releasing the lamb.

Black disease or infectious necrotic hepatitis (*4, 10, 12*), is an acute malady affecting mature sheep in good condition. The disease is due to the germ *Clostridium novyi* type B (*Cl. oedematiens*) in the presence of liver flukes, and it may occur wherever flukes are present, which is usually on swampy, poorly drained land. Black disease is most prevalent in the late summer and early fall.

The onset of the disease is sudden and acute. The first evidence of the existence of the malady in a flock is usually the finding of dead sheep in the morning, although everything appeared to be in order the night before when the animals were penned or bedded down. The dead animals show no evidence of having struggled and appear as though they had died in their sleep. Bloody foam may come from the nose. If the flock is closely watched, stragglers may be observed lagging behind the rest of the flock or lying down instead of feeding. When aroused, such an animal will quickly start away, only to stop and stand quietly or lie down again after having rejoined the band. There may or may not be modaerate fever and slightly increased respiration. Death may occur within an hour after these symptoms are first seen. Because of the difficulty of recognizing the disease from the symptoms alone, it is not known whether affected animals ever recover, but the mortality is probably very high and recovery rare.

At autopsy, if the animal has not been dead too long, a peculiar sweetish odour may be detected on opening the carcass. This will not in evidence if post mortem decomposition and bloating have taken place. When affected animals are skinned, the inner surface of the pelt usually has a blackish appearance, from which the common name "black disease" arises. Since the discolouration is due to congestion of the skin, it is not necessarily characteristic of black disease only but may be observed in one form or another in other diseases. The lungs, though sometimes slightly congested, are usually essentially normal. The lung and peritoneal cavities and the heart sac usually contain considerable quantities of clear straw-coloured or slightly blood-tinged fluid. Some of this may become clotted or congealed, forming jellylike masses. Small hemorrhages may be present on the inner surfaces of the heart. The liver is thickened, darkened, and friable and contains one to many areas of necrosis, grayish yellow in colour and varying from one-fourth inch to an inch or more in diameter. Hemorrhages beneath the liver capsule and minute punctures of the capsule by young flukes may be found. Numerous very small flukes may be found in the liver tissue, but full-grown flukes are seldom present in this disease. The inner lining of the fourth stomach, or abomasum, is frequently slightly inflamed, being of a deep pink colour. If examination of a sheep that has just died in a region where liver flukes abound discloses the lesions described, black disease may be strongly suspected. Effective post mortem examination of sheep can be made only if decomposition and bloating have not reached an advanced stage. If decomposition is marked, the changes due to disease may be somewhat, if not entirely, obscured. Post mortem examination of several dead animals is frequently desired by the veterinarian, and laboratory examination may be advisable.

Clostridium novyi apparently does not of itself produce black disease; initial damage to the liver by flukes is required before the organism increases and forms its death-dealing toxin. Hence, control of liver flukes is of primary importance in preventing the disease. Treatment of sheep with carbon tetrachloride or other fluke-killing drugs after the germ has grown and produced its toxin in the liver cannot be expected to cure the sheep. Such medication is rather to be considered as part of the basic fluke-control programme, through which black disease can be effectively prevented. Once infectious necrotic hepatitis becomes established in a flock through the agency of acute fluke infestation, there is little that can be done except to move the sheep to fluke-free land. Losses may then continue until the acute stages of the fluke invasion have passed. Other trouble, however, still threatens from chronic fluke infestation and pasture contamination.

Bacterin (anaculture), toxoid, and antitoxin, prepared in the laboratory from cultures of *Clostridium novyi*-type B, have been reported to be of value in the prevention of black disease (*14, 16*). These biological products have not been commonly adopted in this country, perhaps owing to the general use of fluke-control measures.

Caseous lymphadenitis, sometimes called pseudotuberculosis, is a widespread chronic infectious disease of sheep and goats caused by *Corynebacterium ovis* (Preisz-Nocard bacillus). The germ is a very resistant organism, capable of surviving for months in the dust of barns, shearing sheds, and corrals. Infection may take place through contaminated feed, inhalation of contaminated dust, or wounds.

The disease affects the body lymph nodes chiefly but may invade the lungs or other organs, depending upon the route by which the infection is acquired and the length of time the animal has been affected. Greenish-yellow or gray cheeselike, pasty, or sandlike pus is formed in the affected organs. In some cases the lesions resemble those of tuberculosis, actinomycosis, coccidioidomycosis, and other granulomatous diseases (characterized by tumor-like formations).

In the early stages of the infection, the animal appears not to be materially affected. Indeed, disturbance of general health does not often come before the time for discarding the animals as breeders. Then progressive loss of flesh and weakness, finally leading to death from exhaustion, may occur.

There is no practical method of treatment of the disease. On first thought it would appear to be an insignificant ailment, but considerable numbers of seriously affected sheep are condemned on account of it under meat-inspection regulations. Moreover, species other than sheep and goats are affected, including cattle, horses, rodents, and even certain wild animals.

Prevention of the disease is promoted by general sanitation and by special care when shearing, docking, castrating, or earmarking. Animals discharging pus from the abscesses of pseudotuberculosis should be isolated, care being taken to dispose of the discharges properly.

Dysentery consists in the frequent passage of liquid feces with varying amounts of blood and mucus owing to inflammation of the bowels. Aside from parasitic dysentery, the disease appears chiefly in three forms, paratyphoid dysentery, lamb dysentery, and Johne's disease, or paratuberculosis, each of which will be considered separately.

Paratyphoid dysentery (7) is comparatively rare, having been reported in this country in a few instances only, in lambs after shipment from the range to feed lots. It is caused by the germ *Salmonella aertrycke,* which is believed by some authorities to be a normal inhabitant of the bowel of some sheep, producing disease only when the animals have been long deprived of feed.

Affected animals are depressed and refuse feed; there is some fever, and the feces become watery and sometimes bloody. Death may come quickly after slight scouring, or profuse dysentery may develop, in which case the illness lasts longer. Losses in three reported outbreaks in the last decade ranged from 2 percent to about 7 percent (7).

In the opinion of some who have studied it, animals kept in good condition and fed regularly during transit should not develop serious cases of the disease. Accordingly, it is recommended that preparations be made to feed sheep at as frequent and regular intervals as possible during transit. If the disease develops, affected animals should be immediately segregated from the well ones. A laxative such as castor oil may be given, and this may be followed by intestinal medicaments and general stimulants. A light but nutritious diet should be provided during convalescence.

Lamb dysentery, sometimes called white scours, is a disease of the newborn that occurs within 48 hours or sometimes as long as a week after birth, the lambs meanwhile appearing normal. There is a very fluid, grayish diarrhoea with an offensive odour, accompanied by great depression, and the lambs stop nursing. Many lambs die within 24 to 48 hours after the first symptoms appear, but those surviving this period may slowly recover. In severe outbreaks 20 to 40 percent of the lamb crop may die.

The disease is essentially filth-borne, and is attributed to several factors, including the micro-organisms known as *Clostridium welchii* and *Escherichia communior* (*5*, *6*). Cold, wet, stormy weather during which lambing must take place in barns and sheds is conducive to the disease if the shelters have been allowed to become filthy. Such places must be frequently cleaned and freshly rebedded with clean bedding if danger of lamb dysentery is to be avoided. Some operators use elevated slatted floors with no bedding in lambing shelters. On warm sunny days, lambing may better be carried out on clean pasture or range. Tagging of the ewes–clipping the long wool from about the udder and the inside of the thighs to provide cleanly conditions for the nursing lamb–before lambing is recommended.

It is often impractical to treat lambs affected with lamb dysentery. Medicinal treatment is usually of no avail. In England anti-lamb-dysentery serum is sometimes used, but neither this nor the other biological products commonly used there with reported success have been generally adopted in the United States. Cultured milk, which consists of sterilized, skimmed cow's milk seeded with *Lactobacillus acidophilus*, has been used with reported success as a treatment by some investigators (*11*). Acidophilus milk can be properly prepared only in the laboratory, and its use is preferably, if not necessarily, undertaken with a veterinarian's supervision.

Johne's disease, or paratuberculosis, is a chronic disease caused by *Mycobacterium paratuberculosis*. This infection causes a chronic inflammation of the intestines, leading to dysentery and gradual weakening and loss of weight. The disease may be fatal in a few weeks or months, or it may be more prolonged.

Exact diagnosis is made through application of johnin, a biological product resembling tuberculin, or through finding the organisms in the feces or tissues in the laboratory.

As with cattle, it is recommended that affected animals be slaughtered under veterinary supervision. Animals suspected of having Johne's disease should be isolated pending diagnosis. After their removal from the flock, pens, sheds, and troughs used by them should be thoroughly cleaned and disinfected. Contact between cattle and sheep should be prohibited. Repeated testing of the flock and the slaughter of reacting animals are usually necessary before the disease is eliminated.

Necrobacillosis consists in the invasion of the body by *Actinomyces necrophorus* (the necrosis bacillus). This organism is capable of producing disease in many species, including man. In sheep, it is of chief importance in sore mouth, venereal infection, navel infection, and foot rot. So far as is known, the organism is incapable of penetrating normal tissues, but once it has gained entrance through lesions caused by a virus or other infection, or through external accidental wounds, it frequently becomes established in the body. The effect is necrosis, or death, of the invaded tissues. What would ordinarily be a mild or inconsequential process without *Actinomyces necrophorus* becomes a serious disease.

Lambs thus infected through the navel or through sore mouth lesions frequently develop multiple necrotic and abscessed areas in the internal organs that lead to serious illness and in many instances to death. In the same way, secondary infection of lesions of venereal disease, caused primarily by a filtrable virus, leads to serious complications resulting in death or an extended convalescence.

Though not a very resistant organism in the ordinary sense, *Actinomyces necrophorus* appears to be able to survive for months in poorly drained, wet, filthy corrals and barns. Its elimination requires drainage, exposure to air and sunshine, and thorough cleaning and disinfection. These constitute the principles accepted as the basis for prevention of necrobacillosis.

The treatment of affected cases is often unsatisfactory. If the foci of infection are so located in the body as to permit exposure to the direct action of antiseptics, recovery may be effected. Otherwise little can be done aside from systemic nonspecific medication, which is generally unsuccessful.

Wound infections in the aggregate cause an enormous loss, which could be largely prevented. Castrating, docking, and earmarking involve surgical wounds, and wounds commonly occur when shearing is done too hurriedly or in a careless manner. The rupturing of the umbilical cord at birth, severing the lamb or kid from the blood supply of its dam, creates a wound that is particularly open to infection. Dog bites and other accidental wounds also provide entrance for disease-producing germs.

Many germs, such as *Staphylococcus*, *Streptoccoccus*, and other pus-producing organisms, may be considered as everywhere present. *Clostridium chauvoei*, the cause of blackleg in cattle and in sheep, persists, in spore form, for years in certain sections and on individual farms. Other germs of the genus *Clostridium*, such as *Cl. septicum*, the cause of malignant edema, *Cl. tetani*, the cause of tetanus, or lockjaw, and others that produce gas gangrene, are more or less widely distributed and are potential killers of sheep. All these and various other micro-organisms may cause trouble through wound infection.

The emphasis here is on the fact that wounds should be prevented as far as possible and accidental wounds should be properly cared for. Even castration can be performed without causing a wound in the external tissues by means of the so-called Burdizzo forceps, or emasculatome. This technique is preferred for that reason alone by many operators. The chief drawback is that it requires judgment and experience that not everyone has. Also, the emasculatome must be precisely constructed for uniform results. Ordinary castration, involving incision and the removal of the testicles, as well as docking and earmarking, should be considered as a surgical procedure requiring cleanliness and the use of sterile instruments. Docking may preferably be done with a hot iron. In all cases, lambs are much less likely to contract infection through operative wounds if, weather permitting, they are afterward turned out to pasture or range instead of being kept in a corral or barn. Shearing can be so humanely done that cuts and scratches are rare. When they occur, they should be immediately touched with tincture of iodine or some other suitable antiseptic. Shearers might well be required to clean and dip their clippers into 3-percent compound cresol solution or some other disinfectant before starting on another sheep. If dipping is planned after shearing, it is best to wait a few days to give wounds and scratches time to heal.

The symptoms that develop following wound infection depend upon the type of organism involved. Pus-forming organisms may become localized or may cause septicemia or pyemia (blood poisoning). Some germs of the genus *Clostridium* produce so-called gas gangrene infections that are usually fatal. Edema and gas are formed at the site of infection, and death results from toxemia. Tetanus, or lockjaw, results from the formation of toxin by the organism *Cl. tetani.* Symptoms may occur a few days after infection has taken place, but usually the interval is 1 to 2 weeks or longer. By then the wound may have healed externally. The symptoms consist of a stiff, stilted gait with bending of the neck and back to one side or upward or downward. The entire muscular system may become tense, giving the animal a saw-horse appearance.

As indicated, nearly all wound infections can be prevented by hygienic procedures, but on especially heavily infected premises where certain types of infection have previously caused trouble, prevention may be aided by the use of specific bacterins, vaccines, toxoids, or antitoxins. Intelligent use of these depends, of course, upon accurate diagnosis.

Goiter

This is a constitutional disease associated with enlargement of the thyroid glands, which are situated one on either side of the windpipe at its upper extremity near the angle of the jaw. Caused by lack of iodine.

Urinary Calculi (Sand or Gravel)

Concretions (hard lumps) or deposits of mineral salts in the kidneys, ureters, bladder, or urethra sometimes cause considerable death loss. The calculi vary in size and consistency from small sandlike particles to large, rough or smooth rocklike or spongelike formations. The trouble is almost entirely confined to males. In the early stages of their development, these materials cause little or no trouble, but if the condition continues there are uneasiness and frequent urination. Later the animal stands and strains in an effort to urinate, and eventually the condition commonly referred to as water belly develops. The abdomen swells, owing to accumulated fluid in the cavity, the bladder is distended, urine dribbles from the prepuce, and dried salts appear in the wool about the opening. Without relief, death invariably follows.

The cause of the condition is not exactly known, though certain feeds, such as mangels, sugar beet pulp or tops, corn fodder, wheat bran, and linseed or cottonseed meal, especially when given in large amounts, are conducive to the trouble. There is experimental evidence to indicate that lack of vitamin A (*9*) and possibly infection of the urinary tract are responsible in some instances. In some cases, responsibility may be placed on the presence of large amounts of mineral salts in the water supply. Again, scarcity or lack of ready access to water may promote the accumulation of sand or gravel in the urinary tract.

The chemical composition of the concretions appears to depend partly upon the mineral constituents of the feed and water. Thus they may be comprised chiefly of phosphates, oxalates, or other ingredients which may be modified by internal medication or change of diet; but this or any other treatment is seldom practicable. In some instances in weathers or rams, in the beginning of the trouble, the small wormlike appendage (processus urethrae) at the end of the penis may be removed, thus permitting passage of the obstruction. Some cases may be relieved by passage of a catheter or sound to dislodge the stones. Finally, the special value of some animals may warrant a surgical operation for removal of the concretions from the urethra. Often, however, serious trouble from calculi does not develop until near the end of the fattening period, and the lambs may be continued on full feed without too serious loss for the short time remaining before they are finally finished.

Stiff Lambs (White-Muscle Disease)

The term "stiff lambs" is commonly applied by sheepmen to any condition causing lameness, paralysis, or a similar abnormality without distinction as to cause, such as arthritis, listerellosis, or tetanus. As here used, the term is given to a specific disease of unknown cause characterized by a peculiar degeneration of the muscles that occurs usually in lambs 3 to 10 weeks old. It is generally agreed that the disease is not infectious. Nutritional deficiencies and autointoxication have been suspected. The disease appears usually among winter or early spring lambs, which because of inclement weather and other conditions are often somewhat confined and restricted in diet. It seldom if ever occurs in lambs born and run on the range.

Although there is no known successful treatment, the trouble can be prevented to some extent by proper feeding and management, including provision for exercise and supplying feed for the ewes that satisfies nutritional requirements, especially as to minerals and vitamins. Diagnosis of the disease is best made through post mortem examination, which reveals characteristic white or grayish streaks in the muscles–those of the legs especially.

Wool and Dirt Eating

Young, nursing lambs sometimes eat wool, litter, soil, and other more or less indigestible substances that may lead to the formation of balls of wool or other material in the stomach. The foreign substances lead to indigestion, and, in many cases, to death, through stoppage of the exit from the stomach. Toxins are absorbed from the digestive tract, and the lambs show stupor, cease eating, and usually die within a few days.

In some cases the habit of eating indigestible substances such as wool may be attributed, at least in part, to close confinement and idleness, but field observations generally indicate that the basic cause of the trouble is a depraved appetite caused by lack of necessary minerals, especially phosphorus. The lambs thus instinctively nibble on anything at their disposal. To provide the needed substances, nutritious green pasture may be provided, and sometimes ground grain or bran may be placed in troughs in creeps readily accessible to the lambs.

Treatment is generally ineffectual, since intoxication due to stoppage of the digestive tract has usually progressed considerably before marked symptoms are observed. The indications are, however, that the trouble can be forestalled in most instances by feeding the ewes a well-balanced ration during gestation and the nursing period.

Literature Cited

(1) BENNETTS, H.W. (1932). INFECTIOUS ENTERO-TOXEMIA (THE SO-CALLED BRAXYLIKE DISEASE) OF SHEEP IN WESTERN AUSTRALIA. Austral. Council Sci. & Indus. Res. Bul. 57, 72 pp., illus.

(2) BOUGHTON, I.B., and HARDY, W.T. (1941). INFECTIOUS ENTERO-TOXEMIA (MILK COLIC) OF LAMBS AND KIDS. Tex. Agr. Expt. Sta. Bul. 598, 20 pp., illus.

(3) BULL, L.B. (1929). DERMATOMYCOSIS OF THE SHEEP (LUMPY OR MATTED WOOL) DUE TO ACTINOMYCES. DERMATONOMUS. (N. SP.). Austral. Jour. Expt. Biol. and Med. Sci. 6. [301]-314, illus.

(4) DODD, SYDNEY (1921). THE ETIOLOGY OF BLACK DISEASE. Jour. Compar. Path. and Ther. 34: 1-26, illus.

(5) GAIGER, S.H., and DALLING, THOMAS (1923). BACILLARY DYSENTERY IN LAMBS. Jour. Compar. Path. and Ther. 36: 120-125.

(6) MARSH, H., and TUNNICLIFF, E.A. (1938). DYSENTERY OF NEW-BORN LAMBS. Mont. Agr. Expt. Sta. Bul. 361, 42 pp.

(7) NEWSOM, I.E., and THORP, FRANK (1938). LAMB DISEASES IN COLORADO FEED LOTS. Colo. Agr. Expt. Sta. Bul. 448, 42 pp., illus.

(8) _____and THORP, FRANK, JR. (1938). THE TOXICITY OF INTESTINAL FILTRATES FROM LAMBS DEAD OF OVER-EATING. Amer. Vet. Med. Assoc. Jour. 93: 165-167.

(9) SCHMIDT, H. (1941). VITAMIN A DEFICIENCIES IN RUMINANTS. Amer. Jour. Vet. Res. 2: 373-389, illus.

(10) SCOTT, JOSEPH P., TURNER, A.W., and VAWTER, L.R. (1934). GAS EDEMA DISEASES. 12th Internatl. Vet. Cong. Proc. 2: 168-187.

(11) SHAW, J.N., and MUTH, O.H. (1937). THE USE OF ACIDOPHILUS MILK IN THE TREATMENT OF DYSENTERY OF YOUNG ANIMALS. Amer. Vet. Med. Assoc. Jour. 90: 171-175.

(12) _____MUTH, O.H., and SEGHETTI, L. (1939). BLACK DISEASE. Oreg. Agr. Expt. Sta. Bul. 360, 18 pp., illus.

(13) _____MUTH, O. H., and SEGHETTI, L. (1939). PULPY KIDNEY DISEASE IN OREGON LAMBS (INFECTIOUS ENTERO-TOXEMIA). Oreg. Agr. Expt. Sta. Bul. 367, 17 pp., illus.

(14) TUNNICLIFF, E.A. and MARSH, H. (1939). AN ALUM-PRECIPITATED TOXOID AS AN IMMUNIZING AGENT AGAINST INFECTIOUS NECROTIC HEPATITIS (BLACK DISEASE) IN SHEEP. Amer. Vet. Med. Assoc. Jour. 94: 98-110.

(15) _____and MATISHECK, PETER H. (1941). A FILTERABLE VIRUS DEMONSTRATED TO BE THE INFECTIVE AGENT IN OVINE BALANO-POSTHITIS. Science 94: 283-284.

(16) TURNER, A.W. (1930). BLACK DISEASE (INFECTIOUS NECROTIC HEPATITIS) OF SHEEP IN AUSTRALIA. Austral. Council Sci. & Indus. Res. Bul. 46, 141 pp., illus.

Chapter 4

INTERNAL PARASITES OF SHEEP AND GOATS

G. Dikmans & D.A. Shorb[1]

[1] *G. Dikmans is Parasitologist and D.A. Shorb is Assistant Parasitologist, Zoological Division, Bureau of Animal Industry.*

As every sheepman knows, internal parasites are one of the greatest hazards in sheep production, and the problem of control is a difficult one. Here is a discussion of some 40 of these parasites, including life histories, symptoms of infestation, medicinal treatment, and preventive measures.

While sheep, like other farm animals, suffer from various infectious and noninfectious diseases, the most serious losses, especially in farm flocks, are due to internal parasites. These losses result not so much from deaths from gross parasitism, although fatalities are not infrequent, as from loss of condition, unthriftiness, anemia, and other effects. Devastating and spectacular losses, such as were formerly caused among swine by hog cholera, among cattle by anthrax, and among horses by encephalomyelitis, seldom occur among sheep. Losses due to parasites are much less sensational, but they are constant, and especially in farm flocks they far exceed those due to bacterial diseases. They are difficult to evaluate, however, and do not as a rule receive the attention they deserve.

The principal internal parasites of sheep and goats are roundworms, tapeworms, flukes, and protozoa. Their scientific and common names and their locations in the host are given in Table 1.

Table 1: Principal internal parasites of sheep and goats and their locations in the host animal.

Group and Common Name	*Scientific Name*	*Location in Body of Host Animal*
Nematodes, or Roundworms		
Gullet worms	*Gongylonema pulchrum*	Esophagus and rumen
	G. verrucosum	Abomasum, or fourth stomach
Twisted stomach worm	*Haemonchus contortus*	
Medium stomach worms	*Ostertagia circumcincta*	Do
	O. trifurcata	
Small hairworm	*Trichostrongylus axei*	Do
Hookworm	*Bunostomum trigonocephalum*	Small intestine
	Trichostrongylus colubriformis	
Small hairworms	*T. vitrinus*	Do.
	T. capricola	
	Cooperia curticei	
(1)	*C. oncophora*	Do
	C. pectinata	
	C. punctata	Do
Thread-necked strongyles	*Nematodirus filicollis*	
	N. spathiger	Do
	N. abnormalis	
(1)	Capillaria brevipes	Do
Whipworm	*Trichuris oris*	Cecum and colon
Nodular worm	*Oesophagostomum columbianum*	Do
(1)	*O. venulosum*	Do
Large-mouthed bowel worm	*Chabertia ovina*	Do

Contd...

Table 1–Contd...

Group and Common Name	*Scientific Name*	*Location in Body of Host Animal*
Thread lungworm	*Dictyocaulus filaria*	Trachea, bronchi
Hair lungworm	*Muellerius capillaris*	Lungs
(1)	*Elaeophora schneideri*	Carotid and mesenteric arteries
Eyeworm	*Thelazia californiensis*	Tear ducts
Trematodes, or Flukes		
Common liver fluke	*Fasciola hepatica*	Liver
Large American fluke	*Fascioloides magna*	Do
Rumen flukes	*Cotylophoron cotylophorum*	Rumen or paunch
	Paramphistomum cervi	
Mature Cestodes, or Tapeworms		
Common tapeworms	*Moniezia expansa*	Small intestine
	M. benedeni	
Fringed tapeworm	Thysanosoma actinioides	Bile ducts and small intestine
Immature Cestodes, or Tapeworms (Bladder Worms)		
Thin or long-necked bladder worm	*Cysticercus tenuicollis*	Omentum, mesentery, and liver
Sheep measles	*C. ovis*	Heart and muscles
Gild bladder worm	*Coenurus Kerebralis, or Multiceps multiceps*	Brain and spinal cord
Hydatid, or echinococcus	*Echinococcus granulosus*	Liver and lungs
Protozoa		
Coccidia	*Eimeria* species	Small intestine
Sarcosporidia	*Sarcocystis tenella*	Esophagus and voluntary muscles
(1)	*Globidium gilruthi*	Wall of fourth stomach and small intestine

[1] No common name.

Another internal parasite of sheep, the sheep nasal fly, the grubs of which develop in the nasal passages and head sinuses, is discussed at the end of the article.

Geographical Distribution

While parasites may be found wherever sheep and goats are kept in the United States, they occur with the greatest frequency and are of greatest importance in the farm-flock area as distinguished from the western or range area. The farm-flock area lies roughly east of a line drawn from the western border of North Dakota to the Gulf of Mexico in the vicinity of Corpus Christi, exclusive of South Dakota. According to estimated figures of the Agricultural Marketing Service of the Department of Agriculture for 1940, there are in this area about 14,659,000 stock sheep and lambs, of which 7,255,000, or roughly 50 percent, are found in Ohio, Missouri, Iowa, Kentucky, and Michigan. Parasitism is worst under farm conditions because as a rule sheep in farm flocks remain concentrated on smaller areas for longer periods than under range conditions. The climatic conditions prevailing, in this area are also more favourable for the development of worm eggs on pastures and the maintenance of pasture infection than are those prevailing in the range States.

In addition to the sheep in the farm-flock area, there are, according to Baker (*3*)[2], about 500,000 goats, the majority of them being located in southeastern Georgia, central Tennessee, and southern Missouri.

General Features of Life Cycles

The life histories of all the common roundworms of sheep and goats, with the exception of *Mellerius capillaris, Elaeophora schneideri, Gongylonema pulchrum,* and *G. verrucosum,* which are discussed elsewhere in this article, are direct; that is, no intermediate hosts are required for their development. Tapeworms, flukes, and some of the parasitic protozoa, on the other hand, require intermediate hosts for the completion of their life cycles, details of which will be given separately under the discussions of the particular parasites.

Roundworms reproduce by means of eggs. With the exception of those of lungworms, which hatch in the lungs (the larvae being

---

[2] Italic numbers in parentheses refer to Literature Cited.

discharged with the feces), the eggs of the roundworms parasitic in sheep and goats pass out in the droppings of infected animals. With a few exceptions, which will be noted in the discussion of the parasites to which they apply, the eggs develop on pasture into infective larvae in periods varying from a few days to a few weeks, depending upon conditions of temperature and moisture. In warm weather the eggs hatch in a few hours. If the temperature is below 40° F., the eggs remain dormant; if it is below freezing, the vitality of many of the eggs is eventually destroyed. Dryness also destroys many eggs, while moisture favours their development. The larvae as they hatch from the eggs are very susceptible to freezing and drying. In very warm weather they complete their development in 2 to 4 days, provided enough moisture is present. In cooler weather the time required for development is longer; at temperatures below 70° F., 10 days to several weeks may fie necessary. Neither the eggs ncr larvae in the early stages develop when ingested, or taken into the bcdy, by sheep and goats; only when the larvae have reached the third stage do they become infective to their host. Hence this is known as the infective stage.

In the infective stage the larvae of many different species of these worms migrate to the stalks of grass or to other plants, becoming active whenever the air is saturated with moisture, as from rain, fog, or dew. When the air becomes dry and the moisture evaporates from the grass, the young worms cease their activity, and they resume their migrations only when the air again becomes laden with moisture. Unlike the eggs and the larvae in the early stages, larvae that have developed to the infective stage are able, as a rule, to survive long periods of freezing and dryness. They reach maturity and begin producing eggs about 2 to 6 weeks after they are taken up by their host.

Symptoms and Worm Infection

The general symptoms of worm infection are unthriftiness, loss of weight, diarrhoea, anemia manifested by paleness of the visible mucous membranes of the eyes and mouth, development of potbelly, or enlargement of the abdomen, and often a soft swelling under the jaw, referred to as bottle jaw or poverty jaw. Since animals showing such symptoms are commonly infested with several species of parasites, it is impossible to determine from observation which species are responsible.

Experiments undertaken to determine the effects on sheep and goats of infections with single species of worm parasites have shown that animals infected only with the twisted stomach worm, *Haemonchus contortus*, show a marked anemia, similar to that produced by bleeding, caused by hemorrhage into the stomach. No diarrhoea occurred. Experimental infection with small trichostrongyles, *Trichostrongylus species* (1), produced a marked, and in some cases prolonged, watery diarrhoea. The infected animals appeared gaunt and depressed, showed evidence of abdominal pain, and refused to eat. Animals dying of this infection were emaciated, and the carcasses showed evidence of dehydration, of loss of water, resulting from the continuous diarrhoea. There was little or no evidence of anemia. In Australia the diarrhoea caused by infection with these small trichostrongyles is referred to as black scours because of the dark colour of the feces passed by the infected animals. This black colour, which was not observed in experimentally infected sheep and goats, may be due to the fact that the animals were on pasture or perhaps to blood in the feces resulting from a simultaneous infection with *H. contortus*.

Sheep experimentally infected with *Cooperia curticei*, another member of the group of worms commonly referred to as small intestinal trichostrongyles, did not show any serious clinical effects (2).

Symptoms shown by animals infected with hookworms, *Bunostomum trigonocephalum*, are similar to those generally found in hookworm infection in other animals.

While the twisted stomach worm, *Haemonchus contortus*, is the most common stomach worm of sheep and goats in the eastern half of the United States, the medium stomach worms, *Ostertagia* species, appear to be the most prevalent forms found in some areas in the western part of the country. The symptoms attributed to infection with these worms are the same as those attributed to infection with *H. contortus*, but they do not appear to develop as rapidly or to be quite so marked. Experimental infections with *Ostertagia circumcincta* (51) did not produce any marked clinical symptoms except in some animals to which enormous numbers of infective larvae had been administered.

Symptoms shown by animals infected with nodular worms are diarrhoea, abdominal pain, and loss of flesh. These symptoms occur chiefly during the time that the larvae penetrate into and remain in the wall of the intestine.

Opinions differ as to the effect on sheep and goats of infection with the thread-necked strongyles, *Nematodirus* species. Such experimental evidence as is now available (*29*) appears to indicate that these worms cannot be considered as producing any noticeable symptoms in infected animals.

Experimental infections with *Chabertia ovina* (*13, 28*) indicate that these worms may be responsible for symptoms of severe bloody diarrhoea during their development to adult worms in the host. The effect of infection with adult worms has not been definitely determined.

Protozoa

A large number of protozoa have been reported as parasites of sheep and goats, but only a few of these are known to be harmful. They are all of minute size, too small to be seen with the unaided eye.

Coccidia

A number of species (*7*) of coccidia, all belonging in the genus *Eimeria* but varying greatly in size and certain other characters of form and structure, have been reported as parasites of sheep and goats. They occur in the wall of the small intestine and cause a disease known as coccidiosis.

The resting, or spore, form of these parasites, which is the form usually found in microscopical examination of fecal specimens, is ellipsoidal or ovoid (football-shaped).

The life history of these parasites is very complicated. The resting, or spore, forms, known as oöcysts, pass out of the body with the feces. Under favourable conditions (*8*) four bodies known as sporocysts develop within the oöcyst. Within each sporocyst two sporozoites develop, so that at maturity the oöcyst contains eight sporozoites. This is the infective stage of the parasite. When taken up by a susceptible animal with feed or water, these sporozoites are liberated in the intestine and invade the intestinal wall. The preferred site in which the parasite undergoes its development is in the cells composing the inner lining of the small intestine. Here the parasites multiply, at first asexually and later sexually. At the beginning of an infection the asexual cycle is more prevalent, whereas later the sexual forms are more frequently found. The sexual reproduction results in the formation of oöcysts, which pass out of the body with the feces and, after maturing outside the body, become infective to a new host.

Little is known concerning the occurrence and actual importance of coccidial infection among farm sheep in the United States. Examinations made in 1937 by the Zoological Division of the Bureau of Animal Industry at Beltsville, Md., of over 100 miscellaneous adult ewes and lambs revealed that all of them were infected with coccidia, thus confirming similar observations made in other parts of the country and showing that healthy adult sheep are carriers of coccidia. During this study the course of coccidial infections was followed in 9 spring lambs by means of frequent fecal examinations from shortly after birth through the following several months. All 9 lambs acquired infection early, as shown by heavy oöcyst production beginning during the fifth and sixth weeks of life. In 5 of these animals that were followed until they were 7 months old, the infection remained relatively high for 6 to 8 weeks after the oöcysts first began to appear in the feces, then declined and remained at a low level during the summer months. These apparently heavy infections caused no noticeable inconvenience to the animals other than mild scouring during the first few days of heaviest oöcyst discharge.

It appears likely that as a result of the intimate relationship between young lambs and ewes, all normally reared lambs acquire coccidial infection at an early age from oöcysts discharged by the adult carriers, but as a general rule thrifty, well-nourished lambs survive these early attacks without suffering any ill effects, and the infections do little or no harm to the great majority of the animals.

According to Thorp (*50*), severely affected animals (Fig. 1) become dull and lethargic, lose their appetites, and suffer from diarrhoea, the discharges often becoming bloody. The diarrhoea may continue for several days, and in some animals for several weeks, causing weakness, loss of flesh, and death. Enteritis (inflammation) may be present in both the small and large intestines. The diagnosis rests on the demonstration of coccidia in the feces of affected animals.

The disease as it occurs in feed lots has been described by Thorp (*50*), Deem and Thorp (*15*), and Christensen (*9*). According to these authors virtually all of the lambs are discharging some coccidial

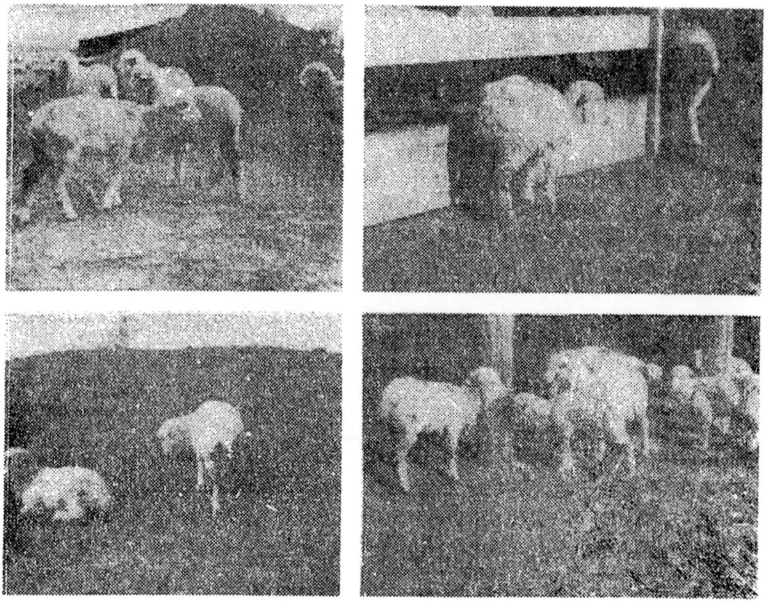

Fig. 1: Sheep affected with coccidiosis.

oöcysts when they arrive at the feed lots. When the conditions are favourable, clinical symptoms of coccidiosis begin to manifest themselves about 2 weeks later. Deem and Thorp (*15*) reported that in a number of outbreaks most of the cases occurred between 2 and 3 weeks after the lambs were placed in the lots.

Christensen (*9*), studying an outbreak of this disease in a group of approximately 16,000 lambs, states that death losses from coccidiosis, together with widespread scouring and heavy oöcyst discharge in the feces, began 12 to 16 days after the lambs had been placed in the feed lots. Heavy death losses continued for about 2 weeks, after which they gradually subsided, but many animals continued to suffer from diarrhoea for several weeks. During this outbreak 540 lambs, constituting 3.4 percent of the total number under observation, died as a result of coccidiosis, and 1,563 required special care and feeding because of emaciation resulting from excessive scouring.

Christensen demonstrated that in the particular case under consideration the source of infection was in the lambs themselves and not in the old, previously contaminated feed lots.

During this investigation Christensen noted that the corn silage that was used as part of the ration became heavily contaminated with sheep feces and that it was customary to replenish the supply in the feed troughs twice a day by adding fresh material to the uneaten portions of the previous feed. No attempt was made to clean out the troughs by removing unconsumed feed, and there was a gradual accumulation of uneaten silage beneath the fresh additions. Whole and fragmented fecal pellets containing coccidial oöcysts were found scattered throughout this silage in the feed troughs. Because of its high moisture content, the oöcysts found favourable conditions for sporulation, or spore production, in the silage.

Christensen concluded that in this case the contaminated corn silage was the principal source of the infective coccidia responsible for the enormously increased numbers of oöcysts found in the lambs 2 weeks after they were placed in the feed lots and for the severe clinical cases of coccidiosis in the group.

Coccidia occur in practically all lambs and sheep examined and under ordinary circumstances apparently cause little or no disturbance. The factors or combination of factors responsible for severe outbreaks of coccidiosis are not well known. The extent to which external factors, such as abrupt changes in feed or sudden marked changes in temperature, influence the development of coccidiosis by lowering the resistance of the animal is not known. Whether in outbreaks in feed lots the ingestion of increased numbers of oöcysts is the principal factor or whether the change of feed is a contributing factor of major importance remains to be determined.

There is no specific treatment for coccidiosis. Christensen (9), however, reports that the daily administration of small amounts of a combined copper sulphate and ferric sulphate solution over a period of 5 weeks from the beginning of confinement in feed lots significantly lowered the discharge of coccidial oöcysts in one group of healthy lambs as compared with that in another group not receiving such treatment. While this test suggests the possibility that there may be some benefit in the use of these chemicals as preventives, there is abundant evidence to indicate that in the actual treatment of the disease, these and other chemicals are of no value.

Globidium Gilruthi

Another protozoan parasite, *Globidium gilruthi*, occurs in the fourth stomach and small intestine of sheep. According to Wenyon (*55*) these parasites, which are probably related to sarcosporidia, occur as sickle-shaped spores enclosed in membranous cysts or sacs, in the wall of the fourth stomach and small intestine. These cysts appear as little white opalescent elevations of the mucous membrane. Within the mature cyst is a mass of spores. One end of the cyst is blunt and the other pointed.

The infection is not uncommon in sheep, but usually only a few cysts are present, and no clinical symptoms or disease condition referable to the infection can be noted. In some cases, however, the infection in heavy, and according to Marsh and Tunnicliff (*33*) such infections may cause a severe enteritis, or intestinal inflammation, manifested by pronounced diarrhoea and accompanied by the usual depression and loss of weight. There is no fever, and no blood appears in the feces except where there is a hemorrhagic condition of the rectum.[3] Since nothing is known of the life history of the parasites, no recommendations for prevention or control can be made, and medicinal treatment has, so far as is known, not been attempted. It is possible that the administration of intestinal astringents such as those used by Christensen (*9*) in outbreaks of coccidiosis may have some beneficial effects.

Flukes

Sheep and goats in the United States may be infested with one or more species of flukes, which are flat, leaflike parasites. Two kinds

---

[3] At post mortem examination of an animal dying from the infection, these authors found the small intestine studded along its entire length with small white cysts, some on the surface of the mucous membrane and others deeply embedded in it. The mucous membrane was hyperemic and had a somewhat furry appearance. In another case the infection was found to be greatest in the posterior portion of the small intestine, the cysts being less than 1 millimeter apart. Microscopic examination of affected areas of the small intestine showed large numbers of *Globidium* cysts, in different stages of development in the mucosa. destruction of the epithelium of the villi, and infiltration of the tissue by large numbers of monocytes and lymphocytes.

of flukes may occur in the liver, and two other kinds are found in the rumen, or paunch. Flukes reproduce by means of eggs, which pass out with the feces and hatch in water, releasing ciliated embryos–that is, embryos equipped with hairlike structures for moving around–known as miracidia. The miracidia penetrate certain species of snails and develop into cercariae (flukes in the larval stage), which leave the snails and encyst on vegetation. Encysted cercariae are ingested by sheep and goats in grazing and develop into mature flukes.

The Common Liver Fluke

The common liver fluke, *Fasciola hepatica*, found in the liver, bile ducts, and gall bladder of sheep and goats is a flattened, leaflike, brown worm, usually about an inch long. There is a sucker on a cone-shaped extension at the anterior, or front, end, and just behind this is a ventral sucker. Through the skin, or cuticula, the branching intestine and the uterus filled with eggs can be seen.

The cercaria, which develops within a snail (Fig. 2), resembles a small fluke and is provided with a tail by means of which it swims about. It finally loses its tail and encysts, or becomes enclosed in a cyst. The encysted cercariae may float about on water or attach themselves to grass blades or other vegetation. When swallowed by sheep or other suitable host animals, the larval flukes, on reaching the small intestine, bore through the wall to the body cavity. Here they wander over the surface of the viscera and walls of the body cavity, finally perforating the capsule of the liver and reaching the extremities of the biliary (bile) ducts. In the liver the young flukes grow to maturity in the larger bile ducts.

The distribution of the common liver fluke is world-wide wherever low, wet pastures and the suitable intermediate snail hosts occur. In the United States it is most prevalent on the west coast and in the Rocky Mountain States, the Southwest, and the Southeast.

The symptoms associated with liver fluke infection are, in a general way, similar to those attributed to other worm infections–unthriftiness, anemia, etc. According to Clunies Ross and Gordon (*12*), in acute cases resulting from massive invasion of the liver by large numbers of young flukes, death may occur after an illness of only a few days and without any symptoms that can be definitely attributed to fluke infection. Sheep suffering from chronic fluke

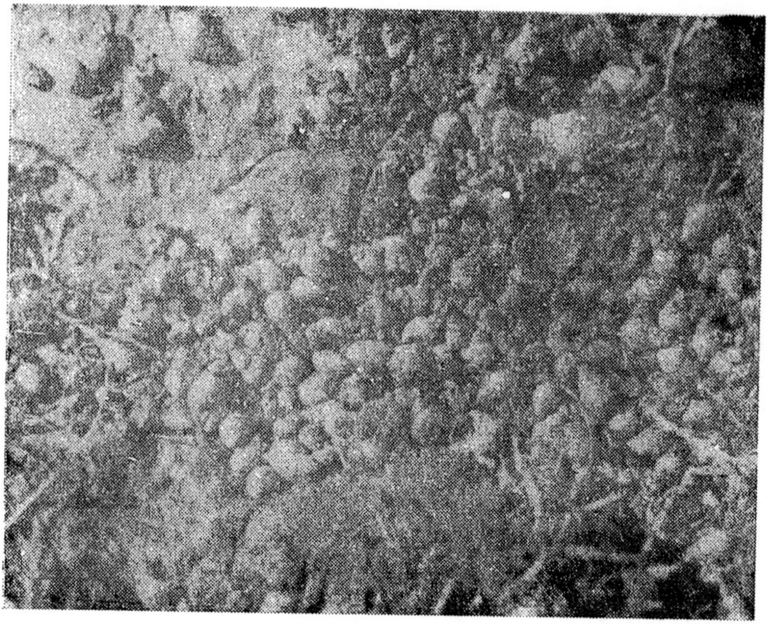

Fig. 2: Snails serve as intermediate hosts of the liver fluke, *Fasciola hepatica.* These snails were on the ground near a temporary pool in a herd pen in Texas. (Photograph by O.W. Olsen, Angleton, Tex).

disease appear languid and are easily fatigued when driven. When such animals are examined the visible mucous membranes will be found to be pale and anemic. As the disease progresses the gait becomes stiff, the loss of condition becomes more marked, and dropsical (edematous) swellings develop under the jaw. According to Shaw and Simms (42), these swellings, commonly called bottle jaw, occur in sheep suffering from infection with immature flukes as well as in those affected with chronic fluke disease. These authors also report that the distention of the abdomen resulting from the accumulation of fluid and commonly referred to as potbelly (Fig. 3) develops during the early stages of the infection when parasites are present in large numbers. The condition later disappears and is not present when the parasites have developed to maturity.

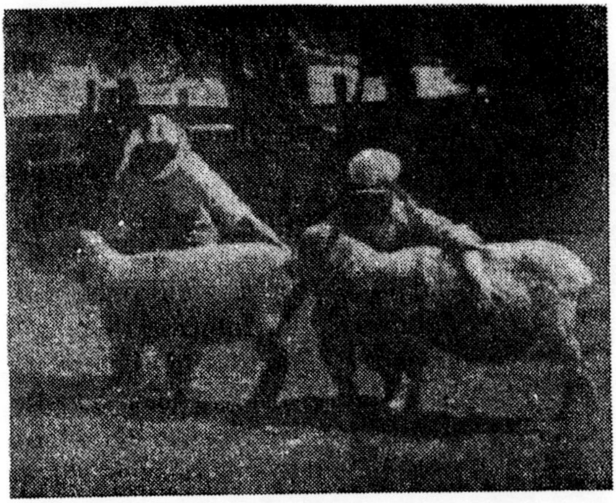

Fig. 3: The sheep on the right shows the distention of the abdomen known as potbelly, resulting from liver fluke infestation. (Photograph by J.N. Shaw).

The lesions found in the sheep at post mortem examination depend upon the developmental stage of the fluke. If the infection is heavy, there is considerable damage to the liver from penetration by the immature flukes. This penetration leads to hemorrhage into the abdominal cavity and an accumulation of fluid within it. Acute inflammatory changes occur in the liver substance, and the liver becomes enlarged owing to engorgement with blood. As already noted, infected animals may die as a result of massive invasion of the liver by young flukes without showing any marked symptoms attributable to fluke infection. After the flukes become mature in the bile ducts, these ducts become greatly thickened as a result of continuous irritation. In advanced cases the ducts stand out prominently and, owing to a deposit of calcium salts, become hard and gritty, as may be observed on cutting them.

The Large Liver Fluke

The large American liver fluke, *Fascioloides magna*, is found in the tissues of the liver, commonly in cysts which usually contain, in addition to the flukes, a quantity of dark-coloured fluid and debris. The fluke may attain a length of 7 centimeters (2¾ inches). The large liver fluke resembles an overgrown specimen of the common liver fluke except that the anterior, or front, sucker is not carried on a distinct cone. The life histories of the two are essentially the same. The same snails serve as intermediate hosts for both, and their development in the snail is the same.

So far as known, deer and sheep are the principal propagators of the large liver fluke. It appears to be indigenous to North America and is principally a parasite of deer, but specimens have been collected from sheep in Montana and Idaho.

According to Swales (*48, 49*), this fluke infects cattle as well as deer and sheep, but in cattle the parasites become encapsulated, or enclosed in a capsule, by the fibrous tissue formed around them through the reaction of the tissues. This prevents undue damage to the liver and the entrance of the eggs into the bile ducts, and it also precludes the continuance of the life cycle of the parasite. In deer a balance appears to have been established between host and parasite, the host reaction being adequate to prevent undue tissue damage but not to prevent reproduction. In sheep severe damage results from the almost unchecked migration of the parasite in the liver tissue. Sheep are the only hosts in which this parasite produces a severe clinical disease. Experimentally infected sheep became greatly emaciated and very weak, even though only a few flukes were found in the liver at post mortem examination.

The symptoms of infestation by the large liver fluke are similar to those associated with infection by the common liver fluke, and the control measures for the latter, discussed later, also apply to the large liver fluke. In addition, however, sheep should be prevented from grazing on snail-infested land occupied by deer.

The Rumen Flukes

Two small flukes, *Paramphistomum cervi* and *Cotylophoron cotylophorum*, one-fifth to one-half inch in length, are found in the rumen, or paunch, usually near the opening into the reticulum, or honeycomb stomach.

The bodies are pinkish when alive. They are convex on the back (dorsally) and slightly concave on the under side (ventrally). Shaped more or less like a cone, they are broad and blunt at the hind end and rather pointed at the front end.

The life history of one of these flukes, *Cotylophoron cotylophorum*, has been studied in detail (5) and found to be essentially the same as that of the common liver fluke, the same snails serving as intermediate hosts of both.

These flukes have been reported from sheep in Australia, South Africa (32), and India, but they occur most commonly in cattle. There is no record of their occurrence in sheep under natural conditions in the United States.

The adult parasites appear to be relatively harmless, and no definite lesions, or tissue injuries, have been ascribed to them. It has been reported, however, that in the immature stages they are definitely disease-producing. The symptoms described are very similar to those of roundworm infestation and the lesions occur chiefly in the small intestine.

Since snails act as intermediate hosts of these parasites,. the methods of prevention later advocated in the case of the liver fluke may prove to be beneficial.

Tapeworms

Sheep and goats in the United States may harbour both adult and larval tapeworms. The adult tapeworm has a head provided with four suckers and a body consisting of a number of flat segments joined together to form a chain. Tapeworms produce eggs of microscopic size which pass out in the feces of the host animal, together with gravid segments (segments containing eggs), which, when dry, liberate more eggs. On being ingested by a suitable host the eggs develop into an intermediate stage–a larva known as a cysticercoid. Sheep and goats become infested by swallowing such larvae.

The larval tapeworms that occur in sheep and goats are commonly known as bladder worms; they are usually located in the tissues or cavities of the body. The bladder worm consists of a head and neck inverted in a membrane containing a clear fluid, the whole structure resembling a bladder. When a bladder worm is eaten by the final host, the head is extruded, or pushed out of the membrane, and passes to the small intestine of the host, where it develops into an adult worm by the growth of segments back of the head.

The Moniezias

Two species of tapeworms, *Moniezia expansa* and *M. benedeni*–long, flat, ribbonlike worms, which sometimes attain a length of several yards and a breadth of three-fourths of an inch--are known to occur in the small intestines of sheep and goats.

The eggs and segments containing eggs pass out with the feces onto the pasture. According to Stunkard (*47*) the eggs contained in the gravid segments are expelled as the segments dry. On the grass of the pasture the eggs are accessible to certain free-living mites known as oribatid mites and also as beetle mites, which serve as intermediate hosts of the tapeworms. The eggs contain six hooked embryos known as oncospheres. In the mite the oncospheres develop into cysticercoids, or tapeworm larvae, in 15 to 16 weeks.[4] Field experiments indicate that during the summer this development may be completed in 6 to 8 weeks.

Large numbers of different species of oribatid mites may occur on pastures, but only a few of these, an belonging in the genus *Galumna* and present on the grass during the cooler parts of the day and on warm, cloudy days, serve as intermediate hosts of the sheep tapeworm. During periods of intense sunlight and when strong, drying winds prevail, the mites leave the grass and are found at the grass roots and in the soil. Saturation of the soil due to heavy or continued rains causes the mites to migrate onto the grass. They may be found throughout the year, but according to Krull (*31*) in the vicinity of Beltsville, Md., they are most abundant during April and May.

The tapeworms of sheep are cosmopolitan in distribution. They are commonly believed to be serious parasites of sheep, and various conditions, such as unthriftiness, loss of weight, anemia, and digestive disturbances manifested by diarrhoea, have been attributed to tapeworm infection. The reasons for this belief are largely indirect but quite obvious. Tapeworm segments are often found singly or in strings of various length in the droppings of sheep running on

---

[4] According to Krull (*31*), the mouth parts of the mites are not adapted to take in the entire tapeworm egg, and the mites therefore break the shell and ingest the oncosphere, which then develops into a cysticercoid in the body cavity.

pastures and showing clinical evidence of parasitic infection. On post mortem examination of such sheep, tapeworms are usually found in the small intestine, and the condition of the animals before death is naturally attributed to the tapeworms. The presence of other parasites, particularly small roundworms, is usually not taken into consideration.

Through experimental infection of lambs with tapeworms (*Moniezia expansa*) only, uncomplicated by roundworm infection such as is commonly found under natural conditions, Shorb (*43, 44*) has shown that the effects of the farmer have been generally overrated. The principal effects observed were a slight intestinal disturbance, manifested by the passage of softened feces instead of the usual formed pellets, and a slight retardation of growth. The severity of the effects depends apparently on the age and size of the infected animal and the number of tapeworms present. Young, undersized lambs from 1 to 3 months of age are more seriously affected by a given number of tapeworms than well-grown, vigorous lambs about 6 months old, and in lambs of comparable ages and sizes those harbouring the greater number of tapeworms showed the more marked effects.

Under natural conditions lambs become infected with tapeworms at an early age, and this infection, added to the roundworm infections usually acquired at the same time, may result in serious retardation of growth.

No recommendations as to prevention can be given until detailed information on the life history of the intermediate host has been obtained.

The Fringed Tapeworm

Another tapeworm, which appears to be confined to range sheep, is known as the fringed tapeworm, *Thysanosoma actinioides*. It derives its common name from the fact that each of the segments has a fringe on its posterior, or rear, border, which distinguishes it from all other tapeworms. If the segments are put in water, the fringes float out and can be easily seen.

The fringed tapeworm is a parasite of western sheep and is found in the East only when sheep shipped from the West are slaughtered at eastern abattoirs.

On post mortem examination of infected animals the tapeworms are found in the small intestine, the bile ducts, the gall bladder, and sometimes the pancreatic duct. At times they may be numerous enough to apparently occlude, or close up, these ducts, and many serious pathological conditions and marked clinical symptoms, based largely on deductions from the post mortem findings, have been attributed to them. After examining a number of infected sheep and comparing their condition with that of similar uninfected sheep, however, Christensen (*10*) came to the conclusion that, at least so far as adult sheep are concerned, no serious effects can be ascribed to this tapeworm.

The life history of the fringed tapeworm is completely unknown, and until it has been ascertained and pure infections have been established, no definite statement concerning its effects on sheep are warranted.

At the present time the most serious loss resulting from infection is due to the fact that under Federal meat-inspection regulations, all sheep livers found on post mortem examination to be infected are condemned as unfit for human consumption.

Bladder Worms

The bladder worms found in sheep and goats, of which there are four kinds, are the larval or immature stages of tapeworms found in dogs and related carnivores. Their names and usual locations are given in Table 1.

Sheep and goats become infected with these bladder worms by ingesting the eggs voided by dogs and related carnivores on pasture or range.

The Thin-Necked Bladder Worm

The thin-necked bladder worm, *Cysticercus tenuicollis,* has the appearance of a large sac filled with clear fluid. A white object, which is the head or neck, projects into it at one end. The bladder is usually about 1 inch in diameter and may attain a length of several inches. The bladder worm proper is surrounded by a cyst wall which is developed by the host animal as a protective measure against the parasite. When this cyst is broken, the parasite usually rolls out and is seen to be a thin-walled structure. By appropriate treatment the head and neck of the tapeworm may be pushed out and made to protrude from one end of the bladder.

When one of these bladder worms is ingested by a dog, the cyst wall is digested, and the tapeworm head and neck passes into the small intestine, where it develops into a mature tapeworm (*Taenia hydatigena*) by the growth of segments back of the neck. Egg-bearing segments develop in 10 to 12 weeks. When infested dogs run over pastures used by sheep and goats they may leave feces containing tapeworm eggs and segments on the pasture, and these eggs may be spread by rain onto the grass and into streams and puddles from which the animals drink. When sheep ingest the eggs the embryo escapes from its shell, makes its way to the liver, and begins to develop. In the course of time it escapes from the liver and becomes attached to the mesenteries or omenta (abdominal membranes). At first it is a bladder without a head, but later a head and neck develop, and the fully formed cysticercus is ready to infect any susceptible dog that eats it.

This parasite is quite generally distributed over the United States. It is most likely to be present where sheep are associated with dogs or where stray dogs commonly run over pastures and where animals are slaughtered on farms or at small country slaughterhouses at which little care is exercised in disposing of the viscera and of diseased portions of the carcasses.

Light infestations produce little damage, but severe ones may make an animal very sick and even cause death. In such cases the animal shows symptoms of dullness, weakness, loss of appetite, and fever. These symptoms are due to hemorrhage from the liver, caused by the wandering larvae, and the peritonitis, or inflammation of the abdominal lining, that results. The symptoms appearing in the early stages of the infestation are seldom associated with the invasion of tapeworm larvae.

On post mortem examination the bladder worms may be found in the liver or in the abdominal cavity attached to the mesenteries or omenta. No particular lesions are associated with light infestations. In animals dying of hemorrhage from the liver and peritonitis resulting from massive invasion, the liver surface shows a series of short ridges or serpentine markings running in all directions and most numerous near the thin edge. On cut sections the liver substance shows many burrows caused by the wandering tapeworm larvae.

Sheep Measles

Cysticercus ovis, the bladder worm responsible for "sheep measles," is most commonly found in the heart or diaphragm but occurs not infrequently in the muscles of mastication and the tongue and sometimes in other locations in the muscular system. It may occur in the lungs, the walls of the esophagus, and the wall of the stomach. This is a small oval bladder worm with the head and neck invaginated about midway between the ends instead of at one end as is the case of other bladder worms. The membrane of the bladder is very thin, with small mammillate projections. Sheep and goats become infected by swallowing the eggs produced by the adult tapeworm in the intestines of dogs and voided together with segments containing eggs, on pastures or elsewhere. After the eggs are swallowed, the shells are digested, and the embryos, armed with six hooks, penetrate through the wall of the intestine and reach the liver with the blood stream. They pass through the liver into the veins and thence to the heart. From the heart they pass by means of the general circulation to those parts of the body in which they are found at post mortem examination. They develop into mature bladder worms in about 2½ to 3 months.

This parasite is more or less generally distributed throughout the western part of the United States and may occur wherever sheep are attended by dogs, particularly where dogs have an opportunity to devour dead sheep. Ransom (*41*) recorded in 1912 that in that year 20,000 sheep carcasses were retained under Federal meat inspection at various abattoirs on account of infection with *Cysticercus ovis.*

No symptoms have been attributed to infection with these parasites, the infection usually being discovered only at the time of slaughter. Ransom records, however, that of six lambs experimentally infected with tapeworm eggs, five died in 13 to 23 days after the eggs had been fed them. The animals died approximately in the order of the size of the doses of tapeworm eggs given, those receiving the smallest doses surviving longest. Three of them received only the eggs contained in a single segment and the other two received 3 and 10 segments respectively. The sheep that survived received only one-half of a segment and was sick for a period corresponding to that during which the embryonic worms were invading the muscles. The nature of the symptoms was not described.

This bladder worm of sheep was formerly considered to be rare, and when it was found, it was confused with the bladder worm of swine, *Cysticercus cellulosae,* the larval form of *Taenia solium,* a tapeworm of man. In accordance with Federal meat inspection regulations governing the disposition of swine carcasses infected with *C. cellulosae,* carcasses and parts of carcasses of sheep found to be infected with muscle cysticerci were condemned as unfit for human consumption. Ransom (*41*) demonstrated that the muscle cysticerci found in sheep were the larvae of *T. ovis,* a tapeworm of dogs not transmissible to man, and he also showed that muscle cysticerci of sheep, instead of being rare, occurred in a large number of sheep slaughtered.

At the present time the parasite is important chiefly from the point of view of meat inspection. Heavily infected carcasses are condemned or rendered into inedible products. The infected portions of a lightly infected carcass are removed and condemned, and the remainder is passed for food. This disposition is made of infected material not because of any danger of human infection but because of the appearance of the meat.

The Gid Bladder Worm

The gid bladder worm, *Coenurus cerebralis,* occurs in the brain or spinal cord of infected animals as a large cyst, or bladder, attaining the size of a hen's egg or larger. It consists of a thin membrane containing a rather large amount of fluid. On the membrane there are a number of small white objects about the size of a grain of wheat, which project into the fluid. These are the tapeworm heads.

Sheep and goats acquire the infection in a manner similar to that described for the other bladder worms–by ingesting the tapeworm eggs voided by infected dogs or related carnivores on pasture or range. The embryos that emerge after the eggshells have been digested make their way through the wall of the intestine and are carried by the blood stream to various parts of the body, but only those that reach the brain or spinal cord are able to complete development, the others dying and degenerating before full larval development has been completed. Those that reach the central nervous system at first move about on or in the brain and spinal cord, forming curving channels. After a while the young worm comes to rest, and the bladder worm develops, completing its development in about 7 to 8 months.

At the time when the young worm gets to the brain there are usually slight symptoms of fever and restlessness, which are easily overlooked. If, as a result of severe infection, the sheep dies at this time, an examination of the brain will show a number of curving channels on its surface. If the infected animal does not die, the symptoms of this stage abate, and there is no further indication of the presence of the parasite until it has grown to the point where the heads form.

Infection with this parasite gives rise to certain characteristic symptoms (Fig. 4), their occurrence and severity depending on the number of worms present. According to Neveu-Lemaire (*38*), animals harbouring 10 to 12 or more parasites in the brain show, shortly after the beginning of the infection, symptoms of depression, somnolence, and loss of appetite and lose flesh rapidly. Disturbances of vision are noted, some animals becoming completely blind and running into object in their path. The visual disturbances are accompanied by disturbances in locomotion. The animals stumble, fall down frequently, settle on the hindquarters or forequarters, and may lie down for whole days as if paralyzed. Death, resulting from acute encephalitis, or brain fever, follows in about a month. There is no evidence of turning or circling disease.

Animals infected with only a few parasites in many cases do not show these early symptoms; in others the symptoms occur, but they are less marked and disappear after about 8 to 10 days. For the next 4 to 6 months the animals show little evidence of infection. After that, disturbances in vision are noted, and they are accompanied by locomotor disturbances manifested by turning movements. The animals walk in circles either to the right or to the left, or they may pivot in one spot; others walk with the head high and with high knee action, or with the head low and a stumbling gait, the character of the movements depending on the location of the cysts in the brain. The animals refuse feed and water and become greatly emaciated. They may move about continuously or stop at times and gaze fixedly at nothing in particular. They are difficult or impossible to herd and tend to lag behind the flock or become lost. When the parasite is located in the spinal cord there is paralysis of

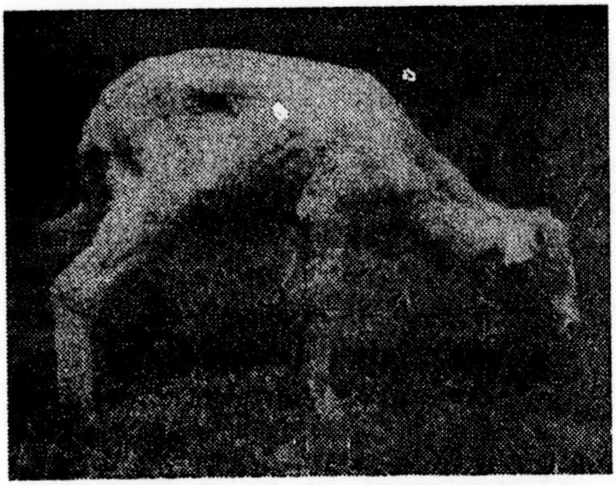

Fig. 4: A "giddy" sheep. (Photograph by M. C. Hall).

the hindquarters, the rectum, and the bladder. At first the hind legs are brought up convulsively; later they drag, and the muscles atrophy.

In sheep that die in the early stages of a massive infection the aborted worms that have lodged at places unfavourable for their development may be detected by the presence in the muscles of sinuous channels, whitish or yellowish in colour and enlarged at one end, where the aborted larvae may be found. Similar tracks, representing the wanderings of the worms, may be found on the brain in 2 to 4 weeks after it is invaded by the parasites. The pressure of the cysts causes atrophy, or wasting away, of the neighbouring nervous tissue and the overlying bone. The bone becomes thin and may even be perforated.

The Hydatid

Hydatids (*Echinococcus granulosus*) occur most frequently in the liver (Fig. 5) and the lungs, but they may be found in practically any organ or tissue. The cysts may vary from less than ¼ inch to more than 6 inches in diameter. They may be single or multiple, sterile or fertile. When located on the surface, the cysts form spherical protuberances. According to Mönnig (*35*) only 8 percent of hydatids in sheep are sterile. When sterile, they contain fluid only; when fertile, they contain minute objects resembling grains of sand attached to the cyst wall or lying unattached in the fluid. These grains are

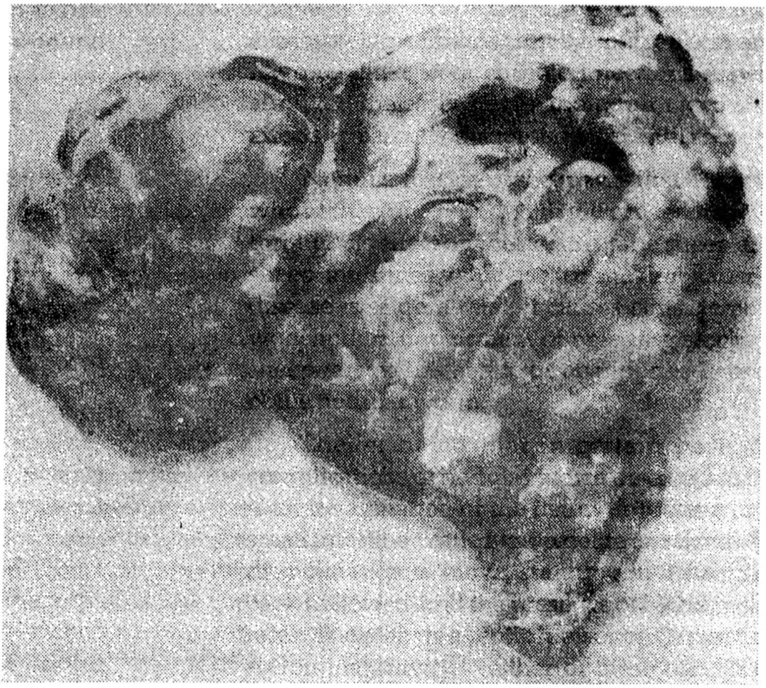

Fig. 5: Liver of sheep showing hydatid infestation.

broad capsules, and each of them may contain a number of very small tapeworm heads.

While this tapeworm of dogs and related carnivores has a worldwide distribution, there is very little definite information on the frequency of its occurrence in dogs and its geographical distribution in the United States. Meat-inspection records covering the period 1930-38, inclusive, indicate that approximately 1,200 cattle livers were condemned each year for hydatid infestation. The locations of the meat-inspection establishments at which these livers were condemned indicate a wide distribution of the parasite throughout the United States.

The symptoms shown by animals affected with hydatids depend on the location of the parasites and their size. If the parasites are small or do not crowd important organs, few or no symptoms will be manifested. When the parasites are located in the heart or brain or some other vital organ, there may be marked symptoms or even death from pressure or from rupture of the cysts. As a rule infestations are not detected or diagnosed during life but are found only on post mortem examination.

Roundworms

Except in areas where liver flukes are prevalent. the roundworms are the most serious parasites of sheep and goats. Roundworm parasites occur in the respiratory tract, all parts of the digestive tract except the second and third stomachs, the circulatory system, and the eye and lachrymal (tear) ducts. The only roundworms occurring in the esophagus, or gullet, and the rumen, or paunch, are species of *Gongylonema,* which occur principally in the lining membranes of these organs and, so far as is known, have no marked harmful effects on their hosts.

Roundworm Parasites of the Abomasum, or Fourth Stomach

The Twisted Stomach Worm

The twisted stomach worm, *Haemonchus contortus,* is the most serious worm parasite of sheep and goats. It is from ¾ to 1½ inches long and about as thick as a pin. The females are larger than the males, and when alive, their bodies are marked with a spiral striping, which is responsible for the common designation, twisted stomach worm. On post mortem examination of animals that have died of stomach worm disease, these parasites are found, sometimes in enormous numbers, in the fourth stomach.

The general facts of the life histories of most of the common roundworms parasitic in the gastrointestinal tracts of sheep and goats have been given. The life history of the stomach worm, *Haemonchus contortus,* as determined by Veglia (*52*), is here presented in detail for the purpose of illustration. Veglia's observations on the influence of temperature and moisture on the development of eggs and larvae of *H. contortus* are also noted.

The eggs are produced in the stomach and pass out with the feces. Under favourable conditions of temperature and moisture they hatch in a few hours, but unfavourable conditions may delay hatching for several days. In the course of the next few days the larvae that develop from the eggs molt twice and are transformed into third-stage or infective, larvae. These third-stage larvae are enclosed in the skin of the second molt and are therefore also known as ensheathed larvae. They do not feed and are quite resistant to unfavourable climatic conditions. When the weather is warm and the grass is wet with rain or dew they climb up on grass blades, with which they are swallowed by host animals in grazing. Shortly after being ingested, they shed the skin of the second molt and reach the fourth stomach of the host animal, where, after another molt, they develop into the fourth larval stage. The fourth molt is completed between the ninth and tenth days after infection, and with the completion of this molt the worms reach the adult stage. They become mature in the course of 2 to 3 weeks. The period required for development, from the time the larvae are swallowed until the adult stage is reached, is variable, but it averages about 15 days. According to Veglia (52) eggs not uncommonly appear in the feces on the fifteenth day after infection, indicating that the adult stage was reached earlier. On the other hand oviposition (depositing of eggs) may be retarded for 10 days or more.

Larvae introduced into sheep by means of water reach the abomasum and there undergo the second molt. Larvae introduced with solid food start the second molt at once, that is, in the mouth. The larvae possess a distinct biotactism, or affinity, for the mucous membrane of the fourth stomach and do not remain in the rumen for any great length of time. After reaching the fourth stomach, they lodge between the minute epithelial processes of the mucous membrane without actually piercing it.

Veglia gives a detailed account conditions affecting the development of the preparasitic, or free-living, stages of *Haemonchus contortus*. The results of his work on the factors of air, temperature, moisture, and light in relation to development and survival of eggs and larvae may be applied to field conditions as follows:

1. Constant warm dry weather, such as occurs during periods of drought, is unfavourable to the development of eggs and larvae of *Haemonchus contortus*.
2. Constant moist or cloudy warm weather is favourable to the development of the eggs and larvae.
3. Constant or prolonged cold wet weather delays development but does not prevent it, provided the moisture is not excessive.
4. Constant dry cold weather, especially if the temperature falls to freezing or below for long uninterrupted periods, kills both eggs and larvae.

5. No definite information can be given as to the effect of variable weather. A very high percentage of eggs and of freshly hatched larvae are killed if during the first 2 days following their deposition on soil the air is dry and warm, provided the soil also is dry. If infected feces are deposited on dry soil, numerous eggs die, even if the first day is cloudy, whereas if the feces are dropped after a heavy rain, numerous eggs survive, especially in grass, even if the first day is sunny and warm.
6. The nature of the soil covering, that is, the pasture and the soil itself, are factors to be considered.
7. The great majority of the eggs passed by infected animals fail to reach maturity.

Various symptoms have been associated with stomach worm (*Haemonchus contortus*) infections, but experimental infection with this worm has demonstrated that the principal symptom is a severe anemia manifested by pallor of the skin and the visible mucous membranes (Fig. 6). According to Clunies Ross and Gordon (*12*), lambs harbouring considerable numbers of worms may exhibit little obvious evidence of ill health provided feed conditions are satisfactory. Even in massive infections no obvious symptoms may be noted for some time, but when the symptoms develop they do so rapidly and are severe. Infected animals become weak, are disinclined to move, and develop the characteristic swelling known as bottle jaw. In animals experimentally infected with the *H. contortus* worms, there was no evidence of diarrhoea, a condition formerly commonly associated with such infection. This has also been noted by Clunies Ross and Gordon, who state that in the great majority of severe cases of stomach worm infection there is no diarrhoea but on the contrary the feces are harder and drier than normal and greatly reduced in quantity. Lambing ewes, ewes with lambs at foot, and older animals may be severely affected, particularly late in the summer and in the fall when pasturage becomes short. Infected animals that show no marked evidence of stomach worm infection as long as they remain relatively quiet may die when driven for any distance. Fat lambs and even adult sheep may die suddenly when heavy infections are rapidly acquired. Such animals may literally bleed to death before they have had time to lose condition.

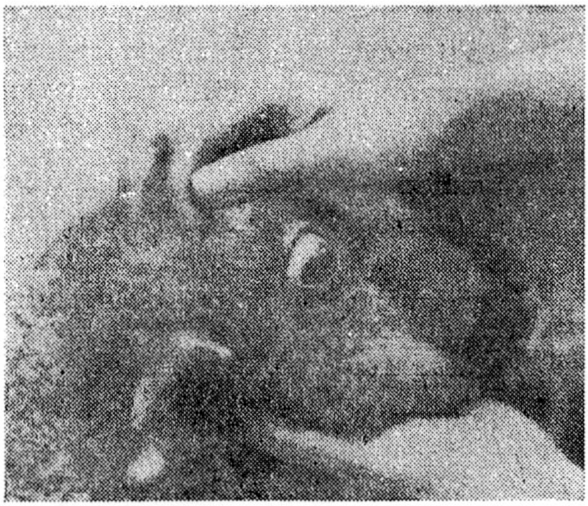

Fig. 6: Eye of a sheep, showing effects of severe experimental stomach worm infestation. (Photograph by J.S. Andrews).

The lesions found in animals dying of stomach infection are those of severe anemia. The blood is thin and watery, and there is a gelatinous infiltration of the omenta and mesenteries. On examination the blood shows marked changes, the number of red cells being greatly reduced. The anemia found in stomach worm infection is due to hemorrhage. There is no evidence that the worms secrete any toxins that affect the sheep adversely (*12*). In experimentally infected animals blood appeared in the feces in 6 to 10 days after the animals were infected, several days before the worms had reached the egg-laying stage.

Roundworm Parasites of the Fourth Stomach and Small Intestine

The Small Trichostrongyles

Sheep and goats are often infected with a number of smaller worms, collectively known as small trichostrongyles, and sometimes suffer severely as a result.

The Medium Stomach Worms, or Brown Hair Worms

The medium stomach worms, *Ostertagia circumcincta* and *O. trifurcata*, are found in the abomasum, or fourth stomach, generally at the end nearest the small intestine. They are small, brownish, hairlike worms about one-half inch long.

The life history of these worms is direct. The eggs are deposited by the female worms in the fourth stomach and pass out with the feces. Under favourable conditions of temperature and moisture they hatch in about a day and infective larvae develop in 5 to 6 days. The infective larvae are taken into the body during grazing, and after reaching the fourth stomach they penetrate into the wall of this organ. Further development to the adult stage takes place in about 15 days, and eggs are found in the manure of infested sheep about 18 days after experimental infection.

As a result of the penetration of the larvae the stomach wall becomes inflamed, dotted with small white elevated areas, and marked with minute hemorrhages. The white spots which contain the worms, increase in size and become nodular–knot like or lumpy–as the worms grow. With maturity the worms emerge from these nodules, which recede and disappear.

Since under natural conditions infestation with *Ostertagia* is usually accompanied by infestation with the common stomach worm, *Haemonchus contortus,* as well as with other worms, it is rather difficult to describe any specific symptoms. Sheep primarily infested with *Ostertagia* species are said to show progressive loss of condition with intermittent diarrhoea and a stunted appearance.

The Small Stomach and Intestinal Worms

Several species of small trichostrongyles (*Trichostrongylus axei, T. colubriformis, T. vitrinus,* and *T. capricola*) are found in the stomach and small intestine of sheep and goats. *T. axei* occurs for the most part in the fourth stomach, while the other three species are generally found in the small intestine, *T. capricola* occurring more frequently in goats than in sheep.

These trichostrongyles are small, hairlike worms about one-fourth to one-third of an inch long. They are usually present in fairly large numbers, but because of their small size they are easily overlooked on post mortem examination. The easiest way to find them is to wash out the first 20 feet of the small intestine in a glass dish and then examine the washings against a dark background. Another method is to scrape the lining of the small intestine and examine the scraping for the worms.

The life history of these small trichostrongyles is essentially similar to that of the common stomach worm, differing only in the resistance of the embryonated eggs (those containing embryos) to drying; they have been shown to be able to survive drying for 15 months under experimental conditions. This is of great importance since it enables the eggs to survive long periods of drought and resume their development as soon as sufficient moisture becomes available, thus continuing pasture infections that might otherwise be terminated by the dry weather.

There are no noticeable gross lesions associated with trichostrongylosis (infection with trichostrongyles). It may be differentiated from haemonchosis (a disease due to infection with *Haemonchus contortus*) as follows: Trichostrongylosis is essentially a slow, protracted disease of young animals, especially lambs and yearlings, which appears shortly after weaning and continues through the summer and the next winter. It is marked by unthriftiness, pronounced diarrhoea (Fig. 7), progressive weakness, and loss of appetite. Anemia is not noticeable at first but becomes evident as the disease progresses; potbelly and bottle jaw are absent in pure infestations. Infection with stomach worms, on the other hand, is a rapidly fatal disease affecting all classes of animals, showing no noticeable stunting or consistent scours-that is, scouring may or may not be present, or it may be intermittent. Anemia appears early in the course of the disease, and potbelly and bottle jaw are commonly present.

Bone weakness, manifested by lameness and spontaneous fracture of the leg bones, especially the femur and the humerus (the upper bones of the hind and front legs), has been reported occasionally in sheep heavily infested with small trichostrongyles.

The Australian workers emphasize that the course of this disease is markedly influenced by the nutritional condition of the animal. Losses from trichostrongylosis occur during the dry summer months when the grass becomes scarce.

The Cooperias

The species of *Cooperia* commonly found in the small intestine of sheep and goats are *C. curticei* and *C. oncophora; C. punctata* and *C. pectinata* have also been reported from sheep, although they occur more commonly in cattle. All of them are relatively small, hairlike

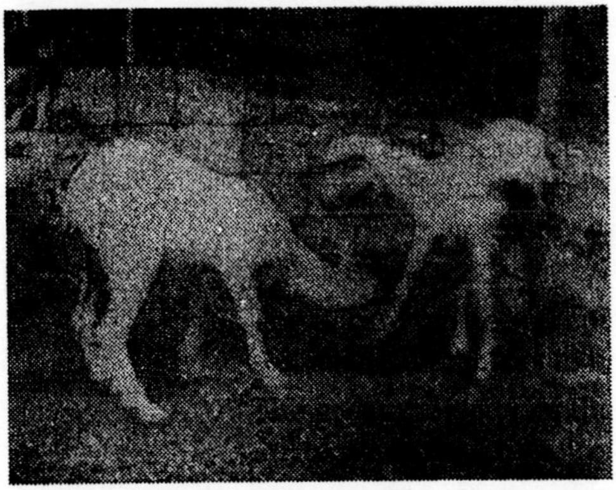

Fig. 7: The thin goat on the right with soiled hindquarters is suffering from trichostrongylosis acquired on an infested pasture. (Photograph by O.J. Hummon).

worms about one-fourth to one-half inch long and of a brownish-red colour when freshly collected.

The preparasitic stages of these nematodes are similar to those of *Haemonchus contortus* and of trichostrongyles. According to Andrews (2) the infective larvae lose their sheaths soon after being ingested and migrate into the crypts of the mucous membrane of the small intestine about 3 days after entering the host. They do not, however, penetrate into the mucous membrane. They undergo the third molt on the fourth day after entering the host, grow rapidly, and return to the lumen of the intestine on the fifth day. They pass through the fourth molt about the ninth day, and eggs may be found in the feces on the fifteenth day after infection.

Experimental infection with *Cooperia curticei* produced no marked symptoms or lesions in lambs receiving good care and an adequate amount of feed, although fatal infections in young goats by members of the genus *Cooperia* have been reported by Edgar (*18*). Andrews (2) reported that experimental infections with this worm decreased the ability of the infected animals to convert their feed into gain in weight, but no symptoms referable to the worm infection were noted and no lesions were found at post mortem examination.

The Sheep Hookworm

The sheep hookworm, *Bunostomum trigonocephalum*, is a relatively large white worm. The male is about half an inch and the female about three-fourths of an inch to an inch long. The worms are about one-half to three-fourths as thick as an ordinary pin.

The preparasitic, or free-living, stages of this worm are similar to those described for the other strongyle worms, except that the infective larvae, in addition to being able to enter the body by way of the mouth, are also able, according to Beller (*4*) and Ortlepp (*39, 40*), to penetrate the intact skin. Beller reported finding hookworm eggs in the feces of a sheep 17 days, and in those of a goat 15 days, after having applied infective larvae of *Bunostomum trigonocephalum* to the skin.

In 1939, on the basis of his investigations, Ortlepp (*40*) gave a detailed description of the life history of the sheep hookworm, which may be summarized as follows:[5] Under favourable conditions of temperature and moisture the eggs hatch in 24 hours, and the larvae reach the infective stage in 5 days. These larvae can infect sheep either through the mouth or through the skin. When applied to the skin, they penetrate it and are carried, presumably by the blood stream, to the lungs, which they reach in 6 days. They remain in this organ for about 5 days. During this time they grow, pass into the fourth stage, and are provided with a provisional mouth capsule. They molt and migrate from the lungs to the small intestine by way of the esophagus and stomach. They reach the small intestine as fourth-stage larvae about 11 days after infection. About 4 weeks after infection they reach the adult stage, and about 5 weeks later they reach maturity, the females at this time containing segmented eggs.

Ortlepp's experimental results are in agreement with field observations to the effect that mature hookworms do not occur in very young lambs.

---

[5] In a preliminary report (*39*) Ortlepp stated that he was able to infect 24 out of 27 sheep with *Bunostomum trigonocephalum* by placing infective larvae of this hookworm on the skin behind the ear. The worms, however, did not reach the egg-laying stage until 10 weeks after the larvae had been applied. In a sheep infected with hookworms in this way, Ortlepp found at post mortem examination, 8 weeks after infection, only adolescent hookworms; no female having reached the egg-producing stage.

While infections with this worm are usually complicated by the presence of stomach and other worms it may be assumed that it does the same damage as other hookworms. This damage consists in the abstraction of blood from the host and the secretion of a hemolytic substance–one that destroys red corpuscles and prevents coagulation of the blood–which causes prolonged hemorrhage at the point of attachment when the worms move from one point to another. Animals infected with this worm manifest the characteristic anemia and edema generally resulting from hookworm infection and infection with other bloodsucking internal parasites.

The clinical symptoms of hookworm infection are identical for the most part with those of stomach worm infection, namely, anemia, edema, and unthriftiness. A clinical diagnosis that will differentiate one condition from the other is practically impossible.

The Thread-Necked Strongyles

The thread-necked strongyles, *Nematodirus spathiger, N. filicollis,* and *N. abnormalis*, are found in the small intestines of sheep.

The anterior portion of these worms is slenderer than the posterior, and the head and neck are thin and transversely striated, or marked with narrow circular bands. In *Nematodirus spathiger* the male is about three-fifths of an inch and the female about an inch long. These nematodes can be differentiated only by microscopic examination.

Their life history differs in some respects, according to Boulenger (*6*), from that of the other nematodes mentioned. The rather large eggs pass out with the feces, and an embryo develops in them. This embryo, instead of emerging from the shell and molting like the larvae of most other strongyles, molts, twice within the shell. Under the influence of alternate moistening and drying or of temperatures varying from 75° to 90° F., the infective larvae emerge from the shells and, like the larvae of stomach worms, crawl up on blades of grass and enter the body of the host animal with the feed.

According to available information, the distribution of these worms in the United States seems to be largely confined to the central and northern parts of the country.

No symptoms or lesions have been definitely attributed to these worms. Recently reported experiments (*29*) appear to show that these worms are not of any great importance as disease producers, at least so far as sheep are concerned, except perhaps when present in very large numbers. Sheep harbouring up to 6,500 adult worms in the small intestine showed no clinical symptoms that could be attributed to infestation with *Nematodirus*, although on post mortem examination minute hemorrhages were found in the mucous membrane of the small intestine at the sites where the worms were found.

Parasites of the Cecum and Colon

The Whipworm

The whipworm *Trichuris ovis* is usually found attached to the wall of the cecum, or blind gut.

The body is made up of a thin anterior and a thick posterior portion. The anterior part may be compared to the lash of a whip and the posterior to the stock or handle; hence the name whipworm. The worms are white, and the eggs are brown and characteristically lemon-shaped.

So far as is known, this worm has a simple life history. An infective embryo develops in the shell, and sheep and goats are infected by swallowing infective eggs in grazing.

There are no well-defined clinical symptoms associated with whipworm infestation in sheep and goats, but it has been found that in man whipworm infection sets up a low-grade inflammation with distinct symptoms of discomfort and distress. In camels a severe whipworm infection has been found to cause a decided thickening of the wall of the cecum with an excessive secretion of mucus, and it is quite possible that in other animals heavily infected with whipworms similar pathological conditions may be produced. The anterior part of the worm is usually found deeply buried in the mucous membrane lining the cecum, or blind gut, and the most common lesions consist of inflamed and thickened areas surrounding the points of attachment.

The Nodular Worm

The adult nodular worm, *Oesophagostomum columbianum,* is found in the cecum and colon of sheep and goats. The larvae are found in nodules in the cecum and large intestine and in heavy infections may be distributed throughout the intestinal tract. The nodular worm, *O. columbianum,* is a fairly large, white worm, about five-eighths of an inch long. The head is usually bent, forming a hook with the rest of the body.

The free-living phase of the life history of this worm is similar to that of the other strongyles inhabiting the digestive tract of sheep.

In lambs a considerable number of the larvae may leave the wall in 5 to 8 days, though some may remain much longer (*53*). In older sheep several months may be spent in the wall of the bowel. When the larvae return to the intestinal cavity they undergo their fourth land final molt and become adults. The first eggs are passed about 40 days after infection. According to Veglia (*54*), the adult worms may live for 21 months, but the majority probably die and pass out of the body in 9 to 12 months.

The chief symptom shown by infected animals during the time that the larvae are invading the wall of the bowel is diarrhoea, the feces containing considerable quantities of mucus. According to South African workers, during this stage infected animals may show evidence of "rekziekte," or stretching disease, manifested by a characteristic position, with the legs, especially the hind legs, extended and the back hollowed. Clunies Ross and Gordon (*12*) report that in the more chronic stages due to adult worms, sheep show progressive weakness with intermittent characteristic diarrhoea containing much mucus. The sheep lose weight, and there is some evidence of anemia.

The larvae cause local injury to the mucous membrane, but in initial infections of lambs in which the larvae remain in the wall of the intestine for only a short while, there is little evidence of nodule formation. In older sheep a more severe local reaction follows the penetration of the wall of the intestine, and marked nodules develop. These nodules at first contain a mass of creamy, greenish material which gradually becomes first cheese-like and later hard and calcareous.

While the nodules, which may extend throughout the length of the intestine, are the most noticeable lesion, it has hot been demonstrated that they are the principal cause of the harmful effects produced by infection with these parasites. It is true that interference with bowel function may result when nodules are large and very numerous, and complete impaction (stoppage due to a hardened mass of material) and intussusception (telescoping of one part over another) may occur when the lumen, or interior, of the bowel is excessively narrowed; but serious effects are reported (*12, 54*) to have resulted from chronic infections in which the animals had survived the early stages and adult worms had developed. These effects apparently do not show up until some months after infection.

Nodular disease of sheep was first described in 1890 by Curtice, who at that time reported that it caused heavy economic losses both through its effect on the health of the sheep and because it rendered sheep intestines valueless for making sausage casings. While the disease is seldom fatal, it causes considerable loss of mutton and wool and an impairment of breeding stock. According to Curtice, sheep raising has had to be abandoned in certain areas on account of the nodular worm.

Theiler noted that in certain parts of South Africa two complications of nodular worm disease are found fairly often. One is an invagination of the ileum (infolding of the last section of the small intestine), called knopziekte or rekziekte, the symptoms being disinclination to move, standing in a stretching position with the back hollowed, and the presence of blood in the feces or stoppage of feces. The other is a septic (poisonous) infection of the peritoneal, or abdominal, cavity. Neither of these conditions is associated with nodular worm disease in the United States.

The Large-Mouthed Bowel Worm

The large-mouthed bowel worm, *Chabertia ovina*, is commonly found in the coiled portion of the colon of sheep and goats. The parasites are relatively large, creamy-white worms, up to three-fourths, of an inch long. They are confined to the Temperate Zone; the records of the Bureau of Animal Industry, in fact, show no specimens collected south of Tennessee.

The development of eggs and larvae to the infective stage is similar to that of other strongyles and trichostrongyles.

According to Clunies Ross and Gordon (*12*), however, eggs and larvae are capable of development at low temperatures; mature larvae will develop even when eggs have been kept continuously at about 40° F. in the refrigerator. After ingestion, the infective larvae migrate to the large bowel, the skin of the second-stage larvae being shed immediately and the third molt taking place after some hours. The fourth-stage larvae have a prominent mouth capsule. The fourth molt is not undergone until nearly 2 months after infection, and the first eggs are not passed until 9 to 10 weeks after infection.

In experimental infections, diarrhoea, often of an irregular character, usually develops about the fourth week, the feces containing much mucus and blood. The growth rate is slowed, and some animals may show extreme weakness and emaciation. As a rule, however, symptoms gradually disappear, and the animals recover after a period of 4 to 6 weeks.

The adult parasites are always associated with visible lesions, the wall of the colon being thickened and edematous or swollen, and the mucous membrane showing patchy congestion and even hemorrhage. According to Clunies Ross and Kauzal (*13*) developing worms may cause even more marked lesions, the colon being congested throughout its length. The immature worms are pinkish, owing to ingested blood. In heavy infections with immature worms there is a definite reduction in hemoglobin and red-cell count, and the white cells tend to increase. The immature worms appear to be more injurious than the adults, but the adults are probably not without effect on the host.

Roundworm Parasites of the Respiratory Tract

Lungworms

In the United States sheep and goats may be infected with two species of lungworms, the thread lungworm, *Dictyocaulus filaria*, and the hair lungworm, *Muellerius capillaris*. Other species of lungworms, belonging in the genus *Protostrongylus*, have been reported as parasites of sheep and goats in other parts of the world, but thus far nematodes of this genus have been found only in deer, mountain sheep, and rabbits in North America.

Thread lungworms are whitish worms up to 4 inches in length. They may be easily seen on opening the air passages of the lungs of infected animals.

The eggs, which already contain embryos when laid, hatch in the lungs. The larvae reach the pharynx, in the upper part of the throat, and may be expelled when the animal coughs or swallowed and passed out with the feces. They molt twice in the course of the next few days, the time varying with the temperature and moisture, and under ordinary circumstances reach the infective stage in about 10 days. According to Clunies Ross and Gordon the infective larvae are not very resistant to drying but are able to develop at relatively low temperatures, that is, about 40° F. After being swallowed by the sheep the larvae bore through the wall of the small intestine and, according to *A. Hobmaier* and *M. Hobmaier* (*24*), pass by way of the lymph stream into the lungs. In 2 to 5 days after infection they are found in large numbers in the mesenteric lymph nodes. Here they undergo the third molt, and the fourth-stage larvae then leave the glands and pass with the lymph stream to the heart and then with the blood to the lungs. They pass through the walls of the alveoli, or air cells, into the larger air passages. Adult male and female worms develop in the lungs about 18 days after infection, and eggs may be produced in 26 days but usually do not appear in less than 5 weeks.

The worms and their eggs and larvae set up an irritation, and the first symptom noted is a cough. While this may occur as early as the sixteenth day after infection (*25, 26, 27*), it usually starts about 30 days after infection and coincides with the development of adult worms in the lungs and the passage of larvae in the droppings. The cough is usually strong and harsh in light infections and may be very soft or even absent in heavy infections (*12*). In severe infections the breathing becomes rapid and shallow owing to the obstruction of the air passages. Heavily infected animals become weak and listless and lose condition rapidly, and death may occur about 2 months after infection. The effects produced by the adult worms, especially when they are numerous, appear to be largely mechanical. The masses of worms and eggs and the exudate, or discharge, produced by the irritated mucous membranes lead to complete blockage of the air passages and the consequent collapse of the lung tissue supplied by them. Large areas of the lungs may thus be rendered functionless, and in massive infections the principal cause of death appears to be suffocation from mechanical blocking of the air passages. The irritation of the small and large bronchial tubes by the worms may lead to bronchitis, which may spread to the lung tissues around the bronchial tubes and give rise to pneumonia. Secondary infection of the collapsed portions also may lead to pneumonia.

In light infections the lesions are usually confined to the lower parts of the lungs.

The hair lungworm, *Muellerius capillaris*, occurs in the small bronchial tubes and in the lung tissue. It is a small, very fine worm, seldom seen against the background of lung tissue in which it occurs.

The eggs are unsegmented when laid but develop and hatch in the lungs. The larva has a characteristic undulating tail with a small spine on the upper side. Larvae either migrate to or are coughed up into the pharynx, where they are swallowed, and then pass out onto the pasture with the feces. They can survive considerable periods of dryness and freezing temperatures in spite of the fact that they have no protective sheath. It has been shown experimentally by the Hobmaiers (23) that these larvae can penetrate and develop to infective larvae in land snails. It is assumed that sheep become infected by ingesting the snails in grazing. After being liberated, the infective larvae reach the lungs in the same manner as the larvae of the thread lungworm, *Dictyocaulus filaria*.

No specific symptoms are attributed to infection with these worms. The presence of the worms and their larvae is indicated by raised, grayish areas on the surface of the lungs. These areas are usually rounded and vary in size from ¼ to 1 inch in diameter. On being cut through, they are seen to be greenish gray owing to the accumulation of eosinophiles (certain white blood corpuscles). At times definite pneumonic changes are associated with these lesions.

Roundworm Parasites of the Eyes of Sheep

Small roundworms, about one-third to four-fifths of an inch in length, may occur in the ducts of the tear glands, between the eye and the lids, or under the nictitating membrane–the so-called third eyelid–of domestic and wild ruminants. These worms belong in the genus *Thelazia*, and one species, *Thelazia californiensis*, has recently been reported as occurring in the eyes of sheep and deer in California.

These worms normally occur in the ducts of the tear glands, but they may escape from their usual location and be found on the surface of the eyeball beneath the lids, under the nictitating membrane, or even in the eyeball. They are white, slender, and tapering at both ends. The males are one-third to one-half and the females one-half to three-fourths of an inch in length. Nothing is known of the life history of the worms, but in view of the fact that a closely related eye worm of chickens requires an insect intermediate host in its life cycle and that putting larvae of *Thelazia callipaeda*, an eye worm of the dog, directly into the eye of a dog failed to produce an infection (19), it is assumed that the life history of the eye worm of sheep also is indirect and that an intermediate host is required in its life cycle.

According to Stewart (*46*) excessive watering of the eyes, or lachrymation, engorgement of the blood vessels of the membranes and of the eyeball, and small areas of hemorrhage on the membranes and under surface of the lids were observed in infected sheep in California. The author notes, however, that some of these symptoms may have been due to infectious keratitis, or inflammation of the cornea, with which some animals in the flocks examined were affected. In other animals from which these worms have been reported, it has been found that they cause irritation of the conjunctiva, profuse lachrymation, sensitiveness to light, and cloudiness, followed later by definite opacity, of the cornea. As a result of invasion by pus-producing organisms the cornea may become ulcerated, and this in turn may lead to an inflammation of the iris and other structures of the eye. If the worms are not removed, the eyelids and the nictitating membrane may become swollen, and, owing to the drying of the purulent, or puslike, discharge exuding between the eyelids, the lids stick together. Mechanical injuries due to loss of sight and the fixation of the nictitating membrane, which is unable to function because of its swollen condition, may aggravate the primary difficulty.

The presence of these eye worms may be suspected when one or more animals in a flock show signs of sensitiveness to light with profuse watering of the eyes, or lachrymation. The parasites are most easily food in animals showing the earliest stages of the clinical manifestations, namely, lachrymation with slight opacity of the cornea and little, if any, purulent discharge. The septic, or poisoning, processes due to secondary infection appear to kill off the nematodes, or at least to confine them to the depths of the tear ducts. The worms are not always seen in a cursory examination of the eye, because of their unusual habitat. It is necessary, therefore, to examine the parts thoroughly by exposing the under surface of the nictitating membrane and the eyelids, when the worms can be detected by their active wriggling movements in the lachrymal secretion. They appear to be washed up with the tears from the lachrymal duct, as any manipulation or application of dressings that tends for increase the lachrymal secretions fecilitates the recovery of specimens from infected animals. The instillation into the eye of a few drops of a 1-percent solution of cocaine or other suitable local anesthetic facilitates the examination of the eye. According to Stewart (*46*) this procedure also causes the worms to crawl out of the inner cornea of the eye and makes it easier to remove them.

Until the life history of these worms has been worked out, no preventive or control measures can be recommended.

The treatment consists in the mechanical removal of the worms from the eye. After the worms have been removed the eyes should be treated as in cases of inflammation due to other causes.

Roundworm Parasites of the Circulatory System

The roundworm, *Elaeophora schneideri*, has been found in the arteries (carotid, mesenteric, and iliac) of sheep. It is a slender white worm. The male is about 60 millimeters (2.5 inches) and the female 110 to 120 millimeters (4.5 to 5 inches) long, tapering at both ends.

These roundworms, or nematodes, have been found in sheep in Catron County, N. Mex., and in deer in Utah. Lesions similar to those caused by the microfilariae, the larvae of these nematodes, have been noted in sheep in Arizona and Colorado.

The life history of the worms is not definitely known, but since they are filarids and all filarids require an intermediate host in their life cycles, it is assumed that some arthropod (insect or insectlike animal) acts as their intermediate host.

The adult worms produce no known symptoms in infected animals, but Kemper (*30*) reports that the microfilariae cause a dermatitis, or skin inflammation, usually involving the skin in the region of the poll (Fig. 8) and in a few cases extending forward over the face to the nostrils and lips. Lesions sometimes occur also on the foot used to scratch the head and on the abdomen where the affected foot has come in repeated contact with the skin, perhaps while the sheep was lying down. The lesions are primarily those of a chronic dermatitis with excessive growth of tissue and the formation of numerous small abscesses. The extent of scratching and rubbing, apparently a result of intense itching, more or less determines the ultimate size of the lesion.

The Control of Internal Parasites of Sheep and Goats

As previously noted, the internal parasites of sheep and goats include protozoa, flukes, tapeworms, and roundworms. Control

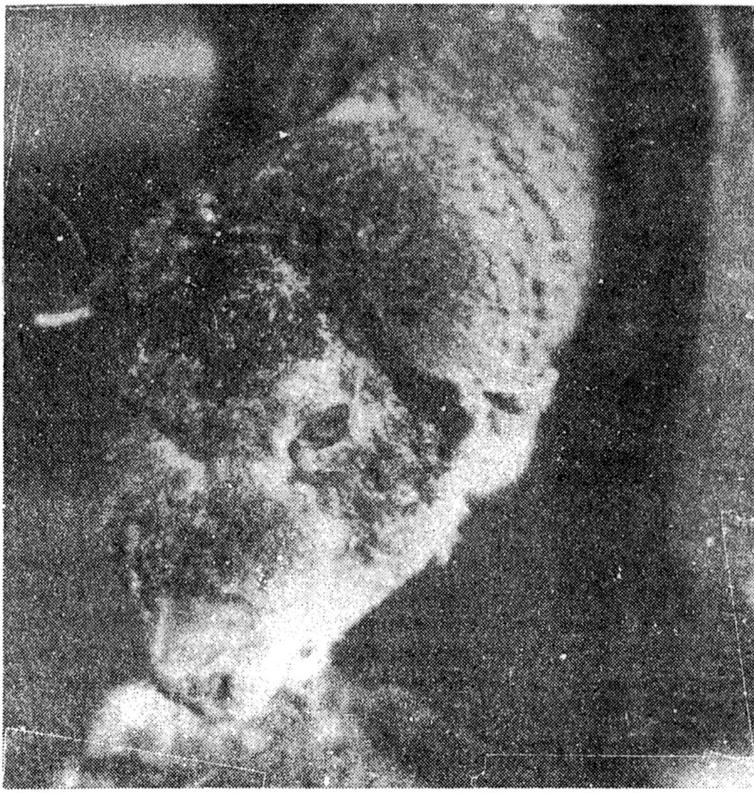

Fig. 8: Head of a sheep, showing lesions caused by microfilariae of *Elaeophora schneideri*. (From Kemper).

depends on effective anthelmintic medication–the use of effective worm medicines–and a thorough knowledge of the life histories of the parasites. There are two phases in the life histories of all of these parasites. One, the reproductive phase, is spent within the body of the sheep, and the other is spent either free in the natural environment of the sheep or in some intermediate host. The intermediate hosts do not serve merely as mechanical carriers, since a definite part of the life history of the parasites is completed within them. A knowledge of the life cycles of the intermediate hosts is generally necessary before effective control measures can be formulated for the parasites that require such hosts.

Control of the Protozoan Parasites

The protozoan parasites of sheep that are known to be of importance in this country are various species of coccidia and *Globidium gilruthi*. They are all microscopic parasites too small to be seen with the naked eye. Seven different species of coccidia have been recently reported by Christensen (7) as parasites of sheep in this country. Whether there is any difference among these species in their effect on sheep is not definitely known at present.

As already pointed out, there is no specific medicinal treatment for coccidiosis. Affected animals should be removed from the flock and isolated, and the exposed but healthy individuals should then be allowed to run over a large acreage to lessen the chances of infection. All straw, litter, or other material soiled by the discharges of affected animals should be burned or disposed of in such a manner as not to form a source of infection for other animals. The premises occupied by infected animals should be thoroughly cleaned and disinfected before being used for healthy animals. In the cases described by Christensen (9), referred to earlier in this article, it is obvious that either some method of feeding should be devised which will prevent the contamination of the feed with sheep feces, or the unconsumed portions of feed should be removed from the feed troughs and the troughs thoroughly cleaned before fresh supplies are placed in them. The extent to which such measures can be applied will depend on the stockman's interest and on, circumstances. Practical methods of using copper sulphate and ferric sulphate mixtures as a means of lowering the level of infection remain to be devised. If, as suggested by Christensen, these substances can be used in powdered form in the feed or in solution in the drinking water and be so distributed as to insure each animal's receiving the required amount, sufficient protection may be afforded to obviate serious outbreaks of the disease.

Control of Flukes

In common with all other flukes, the flukes of sheep and goats require a snail intermediate host for the completion of their life styles. It is obvious, therefore, that the control of these parasites in sheep and goats depends on the control of the snails. A thorough knowledge of the environment, distribution, etc., of the intermediate hosts is necessary to accomplish this control.

The most effective medicinal treatment of sheep and goats for liver fluke infection is the administration of carbon tetrachloride. For convenience in administration, this drug can be incorporated in a suitable vehicle, such as liquid paraffin or raw linseed oil. Carbon tetrachloride, however, is effective only against the adult parasites in the bile ducts. Immature flukes which may be present in the liver tissues or which have only recently arrived in the bile ducts are not affected by the treatment, and it should therefore be repeated at intervals to remove the flukes as they mature. Although the carbon tetrachloride treatment is normally safe for sheep, it may, at times, according to Clunies Ross and Gordon (*12*), be followed by heavy losses 3 to 4 days after the drug has been administered. Affected animals show evidence of acute abdominal pain, and at post mortem examination acute inflammation of the fourth stomach and intestine are noted. Scattered hemorrhages are found in the mesenteries and pleura–the membrane lining the thorax and covering the lung. These authors also report that some sheep lose their wool 2 to 3 weeks after treatment.

While the reasons for this occasional toxicity of carbon tetrachloride for sheep are not well known, certain general precautions should be observed: Only reliable preparations of carbon tetrachloride, free from phosgene and sulphur impurities, should be used; when liquid paraffin is used as a vehicle in the administration of the drug, it should be of a high medicinal quality; where the drug has not previously been employed, a trial group of sheep should be treated a few days ahead of the whole flock; abrupt changes of feed prior to treatment should be avoided; feeding of concentrates should be discontinued at least a week before treatment; sheep should never be drenched in cold, inclement weather; if there is any indication of mineral deficiency, sheep should be given access to mineral supplements containing a mixture of steamed bonemeal and salt and ground limestone or dicalcium phosphate and salt (*12*).

The destruction of the snails[6] which are the hosts of the intermediate stages of the fluke is the most important control measure.

---

[6] For details see: JAY, ROBERT. CONTROL OF LIVER FLUKES AND FLUKE DISEASE OF SHEEP, GOATS, AND CATTLE. U.S. Bur. Anim. Indus. Cir., 6 pp., illus. 1938. (Revised) [Processed].

This may be accomplished by drainage of wet areas where snails propagate, by the use of copper sulphate (bluestone, blue vitriol) for their destruction, or by a combination of the two. Since snails re quire a certain amount of water in which to live and propagate, drainage is the preferred method. Complete drainage so changes the environment as to make it impossible for snails to survive. If the drainage ditches are kept open and clean, the drained area will remain unfavourable for snails and will require no other attention. If the ditches become infested, treating the banks with copper sulphate will destroy the snails. Drainage is not always possible, however, because of the cost or engineering difficulties; though in figuring the cost of any drainage project, the increased value of the land and of the improved forage that can be produced should always be considered. Wherever drainage is either impractical or impossible the treatment of snail-infested areas with copper sulphate should be considered.

Copper sulphate has proved to be very effective for killing snails. While this chemical, diluted 1 part to 1,500,000 parts of water, will kill them overnight, the thorough distribution of such small amounts is difficult to accomplish, and it is usually applied in much greater concentrations.

Copper sulphate kills the snails, the miracidia, and the free-swimming cercariae. It does not injure the fluke eggs or the encysted cercariae; hence, to prevent infestation, the snails should be destroyed before the water and grasses become infected. As used in dilutions for killing snails, copper sulphate is not injurious to grasses or flowering plants and will not poison livestock. It will, however, kill the lower forms of plant life, such as the algae and mosses, and it may kill fish.

The method of application varies with the movement and distribution of the infested waters. In a stream originating on a stockman's land and with the water confined within definite banks, sacks containing large crystals of copper sulphate may be placed in the headwaters. To reach the snails on the banks, dams may be thrown across the stream at various places, depending on the fall of the stream, to raise the treated water to cover the snails. Overflow lands, stagnant backwaters, marshes, pools, and similar wet places are best treated by broadcasting powdered copper sulfate. The water troughs, and especially the puddles around the troughs, should not be overlooked. It is more economical to use the powdered than the crystalline copper sulphate for treating these places. The chemical may be mixed with a carrier such as sand or land plaster in the proportion of 1 part of the copper sulphate to 4 to 8 parts of the carrier, depending on the volume of water to be treated. The land plaster has the advantage of marking the treated area. The airplane has been found to be practical in spreading copper sulphate over large, swampy areas, but when applied in this way the copper sulphate and carrier mixture must be fine enough to be applied as a dust.

To estimate the amount of copper sulphate needed to treat the water in a stream, it is necessary to know the flow in cubic feet per second. To determine this, select a uniform section of the stream about 50 feet long, measure the width and the average depth of the flowing water, and multiply them to get the area of the cross section in square feet. Mark off 50 feet, throw a chip in the water at the upper end, and ascertain the number of seconds required for the chip to float the 50 feet. Divide this by 50 to obtain the velocity in feet per second. The number of square feet of cross section multiplied by the velocity in feet per second equals the approximate flow in cubic feet per second. For example: A stream 6 feet wide has an average depth of 6 inches; the area of cross section equals 6 times 0.5, or 3 square feet. If it takes a chip 25 seconds to float 50 feet, the rate of flow is 2 feet per second. Multiply the cross section (3 square feet) by the velocity (2 feet per second) and the result is a flow of 6 cubic feet per second. For a 24-hour treatment at a dilution of 1 to 500,000 parts of water, 12 pounds of copper sulphate are required for each cubic foot per second of flow. Therefore, the amount of copper sulphate required for this stream would be 6 times 12, or 72 pounds.

Where the amount of copper sulphate required to treat the water in a lake would be excessive or where the lake is used as a fish preserve, the copper sulphate may be broadcast along the banks and on the water a few feet out from the bank.

A few days after treating the water it is well to make a careful investigation of the effect on the snails. Usually one treatment at the right time is enough for a year, but if live snails are found after an application of copper sulfate, the waters should have another application. When once a range is infested, it is necessary to repeat the copper-sulfate treatment once a year until all snails are killed.

The best time to treat is when the greatest number of snails can be reached; usually this is after the spring rains.

Often a combination of drainage and the use of copper sulphate will bring about the desired results. Where complete drainage is either impractical or impossible, partial drainage may prove to be of value in reducing the size of the wet area. The remaining undrained portion can then be treated with copper sulfate. The methods used will depend entirely on local conditions.

Control of Roundworms

Except in the areas where liver flukes occur, the roundworms are the most important parasites of sheep and goats. With the exception of *Elaeophora schneideri*, a threadworm found in the blood vessels of sheep, *Gongylonema pulchrum* and *G. verrucosum* (the gullet worms), and *Muellerius capillaris*, one of the lungworms, the life histories of all the roundworm parasites of sheep are direct, no intermediate hosts being required.

The only known effective method of attacking the parasites in the parasitic phase of their existence consists in anthelmintic medication. Many drugs have been tried and recommended as anthelmintics, but, for all practical purposes, there are at the present time only three drugs and only combination of drugs available for effective treatment: Phenothiazine; copper sulfate, tetrachlorethylene, and a combination of copper sulphate and nicotine solution.

Phenothiazine has a very high degree of efficacy when used in the treatment of sheep for large stomach worms, *Haemonchus contortus*; hookworms, *Bunostomum trigonocephalum*, nodular worms, *Oesophagostomum columbianum*, and large-mouthed bowel worms, *Chabertia ovina*. It has given satisfactory results when used in treating sheep for the small trichostrongyles, *Ostertagia*, *Trichostrongylus*, and *Cooperia* species (Fig. 9, *A* and *B*). It appears to be ineffective, however, in the treatment of sheep for the removal of thread-necked strongyles, *Nematodirus* species; whipworms, *Trichuris* species; and lungworms and tapeworms.

Copper sulphate alone is effective against the common twisted stomach worm, *Haemonochus contortus*, but it is not very effective against the other worms found in the stomach and small intestines. Copper sulphate and nicotine solution, commonly referred to as Cu-Nic, is as effective against the common stomach worm as copper

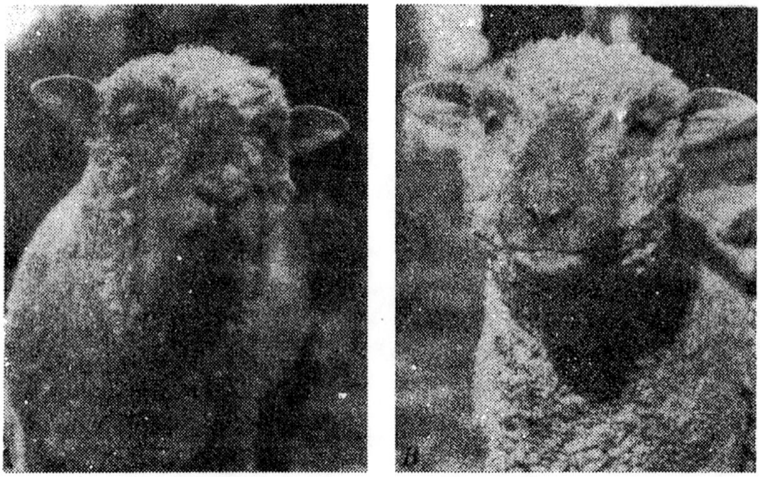

Fig. 9: *A*: Bottle jaw in a sheep suffering from general gastrointestinal parasitism; *B*: the same sheep 19 days after treatment with phenothiazine. (From Habermann and Hunt).

sulphate alone and is more effective than copper sulphate alone against the other worms found in the stomach and against some of the worms in the small intestine. Tetrachlorethylene appears to be effective against stomach and intestinal worms, and it is apparently more effective against the small trichostrongyles than either copper sulphate or a mixture of copper sulphate and nicotine solution. The thread-necked strongyles, *Nematodirus* species, are only slightly affected by treatment. However, so far as is known at present, these parasites do not produce any serious disturbance in sheep in spite of the fact that they may be present in large numbers. The nodular worm, *Oesophagostomum columbianum*, and the large intestinal worm, *Chabertia ovina*, are not amenable to treatment with either Cu-Nic or tetrachlorethylene. South African workers, however, report good results from a treatment consisting of a mixture of copper arsenate, 2 parts; calcium hydroxide, or slaked lime, 3 parts; and copper tartrate, 5 parts. The dose of this mixture is 1 gram (15 grains) for lambs 3 to 6 months old; 1.8 grams (27 grains) for lambs 6 to 18 months old; and 2.5 grams (37.5 grains) for animals over 18 months old. Two doses are given on consecutive days, and each treatment is preceded by the administration of 2.5 cc. of a 10-percent solution of copper sulfate. The treatment is administered as follows: The sheep's mouth is opened wide and the copper sulphate solution is poured alongside the tongue so that it runs down into the throat; then before the sheep's mouth is closed, the proper dose of the copper arsenate, lime, and copper tartrate mixture, which is made up in the form of a powder, is placed on the back of the tongue. The treatment is repeated the next day. Sheep should not be even grain or be permitted access to a salt lick for 2 days before and1 day after the treatment. If the pasture is dry, green feed should be furnished for a few hours before dosing. Sheep must not be kept from feed and water before treatment. After treatment they may graze immediately but should have no water for 1 to 2 hours.

Suckling lambs should not be treated unless this is necessary. If treatment is necessary the lambs should not be permitted access to water from 4 hours before to 4 hours after the treatment. Weak lambs should receive only one dose, and weak sheep and those that are small for their ages should get a smaller dose on the second day.

From this brief review it is quite clear that from the viewpoint of anthelmintic treatment it does not make any great difference with what particular roundworms the sheep are infected. Two things are necessary:

(1) An accurate diagnosis of worm infection should be made, and

(2) Anthelmintic treatment should be given as and when necessary.

The prevention of infection with gastrointestinal roundworms depends upon a thorough knowledge of the preparasitic, or free-living, stages of these parasites–the egg and the first, second, and third (infective) larval stages. As already noted in connection with roundworms in general and *Haemonchus contortus* in particular, the development and survival of these stages depend on conditions of temperature, moisture, soil, sunlight, etc.

Reports of some recent observations on the longevity of infective larvae of various species of parasitic roundworms indicate that the major portion of these larvae died within a few weeks after they were placed on grass plots outdoors and that only a comparatively small number survived for as long as 4 months. Other reports show that the infective larvae of some species may survive much longer. There is a marked difference in the ability of the eggs and infective larvae of the various species to withstand unfavourable environmental conditions, and much more detailed information is necessary before general recommendations for the prevention of parasitic infection applicable to various parts of the United States can be made. Present indications, however, are that the majority of the infective larvae die in periods of 6 to 12 weeks, but since infective larvae develop under favourable conditions in 4 to 10 days after the eggs reach the pasture, it is clear that pasture rotation alone at intervals of 6 weeks and over cannot be relied on to control parasites.

There is no completely satisfactory medicinal treatment for the removal of lungworms from sheep and goats. The intratracheal injection of various drugs and combinations of drugs, the inhalation of chloroform and sulfur fumes, and the administration of certain volatile compounds that are excreted through the lungs, have been recommended by various authors. Clunies Ross and Gordon state that in Australia the intratracheal injection of a mixture of 1 part creosote, 1 part chloroform, 2 parts turpentine, and 4 parts olive oil, in doses of 4 milliliters (1 dram) for lambs, is recommended. In other countries intratracheal injections of pyrethrin in olive oil and Lugol's solution of iodine in glycerine are advocated, but Monnig (*36*) reports that intratracheal injections with the latter two substances are of little value.

The development from eggs to infective larvae can take place through quite a wide range of temperature, and the results of cultural experiments indicate that lungworm larvae are well adapted to temperate climates. Although the infective larvae are quite resistant to unfavourable environmental conditions, the eggs and the first- and second-stage larvae are destroyed by drying, and it is a common observation that lungworm infections by *Dictyocaulus filaria* are intimately connected with low-lying, wet pastures. The use of such areas as pastures, wherever the topography permits of a choice, should therefore be avoided. This applies also, of course, to the prevention of infection with other worm parasites. Removal of lungworm-infected animals from infected pastures to dry lots to avoid constant reinfection is also to be recommended wherever it is practicable.

As previously noted, the gullet worms *Gongylonema pulchrum* and *G. verrucosum*, the hair lungworm *Muellerius capillaris*, and *Elaeophora schneideri*, a roundworm found in the blood vessels of sheep and deer, require intermediate hosts in their life cycles.

There is no medicinal treatment for the removal of either gullet worms or hair lungworms. Kemper (*30*) reports that the administration of fuadin was of benefit in the case of sheep infected with *Elaeophora schneideri*. The administration of 88 cubic centimeters or more of fuadin intramuscularly in doses of 4 cubic centimeters daily was followed by complete healing of the skin lesions caused by the microfilariae of this parasite.

The tapeworms *Moniezia expansa*, *M. benedeni*, and *Thysanosoma actinioides* also require intermediate hosts in their life cycles. The combination of copper sulphate and nicotine solution has been reported as effective for the removal of tapeworms (*Moniezia* spp.) from sheep (*20*), but there is no effective medicinal treatment for the removal of the fringed tapeworm, *Thysanosoma actinioides*.

The prevention of infection with bladder worms obviously consists in the proper disposal of all infected sheep carcasses and parts of carcasses, the elimination of stray dogs, and the examination and proper anthelmintic treatment, whenever necessary, of all dogs that can come in contact with sheep or wander over the pastures on which the sheep graze.

Where sheep are housed during the winter months it is a good practice to treat them once every month in order to reduce the infection to a minimum. When such sheep and their lambs are placed on pasture in the spring, most of the pasture infection will have been eliminated; and, with only a few parasites in the old sheep, it will take some time for a pasture infection to build up to a point where it becomes dangerous. Frequent rotation of pasture, with the sheep not returning to any one pasture in less than 3 months, will be a material aid in controlling infection.

The well-known recommendation for early lambing is based on the known influence of climatic conditions on pasture infection. Low temperatures retard development of eggs and larvae, and temperatures sufficiently low and prolonged will kill them. Lambs dropped early in the season and well cared for will either be ready for market, before the favourable season for parasitic development arrives, or if they are retained for flock replacements, they will be in a better condition to withstand parasitic infection than lambs dropped later in the season and going on pasture when the weather favours development of parasites.

One of the most beneficial results of pasture rotation lies in the improved grazing furnished by the pasture as a result of rest and the consequent improved feeding conditions for the animals. While more information is needed concerning the relation of nutrition to parasitic disease, common observation and such experimental evidence as is available indicate very clearly that the nutritional state of the animal has a decided influence on its susceptibility to parasitic attacks. Clunies Ross and Gordon (*11*) found that resistance to stomach worm infection in older sheep was broken down when the sheep were kept for a considerable time on a diet low in protein and minerals.

The Sheep Nasal Fly

The condition in sheep commonly referred to as grub-in-the-head is due to the larvae or grubs of the sheep nasal fly, *Oestrus ovis,* also called the sheep gadfly and the head maggot fly. This fly is somewhat larger than the common horsefly, dull yellow or brownish in colour, and hairy (*22*).

The flies are active during the warm part of the day and rest in warm corners and crevices during the cooler parts. They are viviparous–that is, they bear living young instead of eggs–and deposit their larvae around the nostrils of sheep. In attempting to deposit the larvae, the flies cause great annoyance to the sheep. The animals stop feeding, become restless, press their noses against the ground or against other sheep, and huddle together under buildings, rock ledges, and shade trees along fences.

After being deposited, the minute larvae migrate into the nasal passages. They remain on the nasal mucous membranes for varying periods of time before migrating to the frontal sinuses, where they complete their development as larvae. The mature larvae then leave the sinuses, return to the nasal passages, and drop to the ground, where they burrow into the soil and pupate. The period of pupation may last from approximately 3 weeks to 2 months, depending on soil temperature and moisture. At the end of this period the adult flies emerge from the pupal cases, crawl to the surface, and become active.

According to Mitchell and Cobbett (*34*), larvae deposited in the nostrils of spring lambs early in the season may complete their development in 2½ to 3½ months. Since such larvae may pupate in 12 to 72 hours after reaching maturity and the period of pupation may last from 17 to 57 days, a full life cycle may be completed in 3 to 5½ months. In New Mexico the flies are active during the late spring, summer, and early fall, and many larvae develop to maturity and are expelled in 25 to 35 days. Many do not develop during the season in which they are deposited, but remain in the nasal chambers throughout the late fall and the winter and do not migrate to the frontal sinuses until the next spring. Cobbett (*14*) expresses the opinion that the flies overwinter in the nasal cavities of sheep as first-stage larvae.

As the larvae crawl about on the nasal mucous membrane they set up an irritation that results in an increased flow of mucus from the nose, resembling that accompanying a cold in the head. This discharge is thin and clear at first, but as a result of bacterial infection, it soon thickens and becomes discoloured, presenting the condition commonly called snotty nose, the most generally recognized symptom of grub infestation. Other symptoms shown by affected animals are frequent sneezing and difficulty in breathing. The eyes become inflamed, and the head is carried low. The animals grate their teeth and lose their appetite, or at least there is interference with feeding.

According to Mitchell and Cobbett (*34*), post mortem examination of the heads of infested sheep shows little pathological change in the tissues affected by live larvae other than increased mucous secretion, even when the head cavities contain many larvae. Only when dead larvae were encountered in the frontal sinus was there evidence of inflammation of the affected tissues, with discolouration and thickening of the mucous membrane and the presence of a thick, discoloured secretion.

Many attempts have been made to treat or to prevent grub infestation of sheep. They may be summarized as follows:

(1) Attempts to kill the grubs in the frontal sinuses of the head by injecting materials through perforations in the frontal bones;

(2) Attempts to kill the grubs by injecting materials into the nasal cavities;

(3) Attempts to remove the grubs by introducing irritants into the nasal passages for the purpose of causing the animal to sneeze and expel the grubs. Efforts to prevent infestation have been largely confined to placing repellents on the nasal openings. Critical examination has shown that the repellents employed thus far are of little or no value.

Stewart (*45*), Du Toit (*16*), and Du Toit and Clark (*17*) report having obtained satisfactory results in treating sheep for grub infestation by injecting various preparations into the frontal sinuses through openings made in the frontal bones. They described the technique of the operation and reported that they observed no deleterious effects from the treatment. They also noted that in sheep slaughtered a few days after the treatment had been given, no dead larvae were found in the sinuses, apparently demonstrating that the treatment completely eliminated grubs from the head. Gildow and Hickman (*21*), Du Toit (*16*), and Monnig and Du Toit (*37*) have described a treatment that consists in the introduction of larvicides into the nasal cavities. The animals to be treated were restrained on their backs with the heads held at an angle of 45 degrees with the ground.

Cobbett (*14*) recently reported having obtained satisfactory results from the injection under pressure into the nasal cavities of a 3-percent solution of a saponified cresol preparation known as saponated solution of cresol. The chief difference between this treatment and those previously described consists in the fact that Cobbett's treatment is mainly directed toward killing the small larvae in the nasal cavities before they reach the sinuses, whereas the purpose of the other treatment is to kill the larvae in the frontal sinuses.

Cobbett reports that irrigation of the nasal mucous membranes of sheep with this solution caused no injury to the animals treated. Some sneezing and coughing occurred immediately after the treatment, but these and the subsequent nasal discharge were of short duration. Occasionally an animal held its breath immediately after treatment and fell to the ground, but such animals recovered promptly when assisted to their feet. The author calls attention to the fact that this treatment is effective as control measure only in areas where the temperature during the winter months is sufficiently low to kill the adult flies and prevent any adult-fly activity.

Literature Cited

(1) ANDREWS, JOHN S. (1939). EXPERIMENTAL TRICHOSTRONGYLOSIS IN SHEEP AND GOATS. Jour. Agr. Res. 58: 761-770, illus.

(2) _____(1939). LIFE HISTORY OF THE NEMATODE COOPERIA CURTICEI, AND DEVELOPMENT OF RESISTANCE IN SHEEP. Jour. Agr. Res. 58: 771-785, illus.

(3) BAKER, O.E. (1939). A GRAPHIC SUMMARY OF FARM ANIMALS AND ANIMAL PRODUCTS. U.S. Dept. Agr. Misc. Pub. 269, 88 pp., illus.

(4) BELLER, K. (1928). INFEKTIONSWEGE UND ENTWICKLUNG DES HAKENWURMS VOM SCHAFE (BUNOSTOMUM TRIGONOCEPHALUM RUD. 1808). Ztschr. f. Infektionskrank., Parasitare Krank. u. Hyg. der Haustiere 32: [232]-251, illus.

(5) BENNETT, HARRY JACKSON (1936). THE LIFE HISTORY OF COTYLOPHORUMI, A TREMATODE FROM RUMINANTS. Ill. Biol. Monog., (n. s.) v. 14, No. 4. 119 pp., illus.

(6) BOULENGER, CHARLES L. (1915). THE LIFE-HISTORY OF NEMATODIRUS FILICOLLIS RUD., A NEMATODE PARASITE OF THE SHEEP'S INTESTINE. Parasitology 8: [133]-155, illus.

(7) CHRISTENSEN, J.F. (1938). SPECIES DIFFERENTIATION IN THE COCCIDIA FROM THE DOMESTIC SHEEP. Jour. Parasitol. 24: 453-467, illus.

(8) _____(1939). SPORULATION AND VIABILITY OF OÖCYSTS OF EIMERIA ARLOINGI FROM THE DOMESTIC SHEEP. Jour. Agr. Res. 59: 527-534.

(9) _____(1940). THE SOURCE AND AVAILABAILITY OF INFECTIVE OÖCYSTS IN AN OUTBREAK OF COCCIDIOSIS IN LAMBS IN NEBRASKA FEEDLOTS. Amer. Jour. Vet. Res. 1: 27-35.

(10) CHRISTENSEN, REED O. (1931). AN ANALYSIS OF REPUTED PATHOGENICITY OF THYSANOSOMA ACTINIOIDES IN ADULT SHEEP. Jour. Agr. Res. 42: 245-249, illus.

(11) CLUNIES ROSS, I., and GORDON, H. McL. (1933). NUTRITIONAL FACTORS AFFECTING RESISTANCE TO HAEMONCHOSIS. Austral. Vet. Jour. 9 (3): 100-107, illus.

(12) CLUNIES Ross, I., and GORDON, B. McL. (1936). THE INTERNAL PARASITES AND PARASITIC DISEASES OF SHEEP; THEIR TREATMENT AND CONTROL. 238 pp., illus. Sydney, Australia.

(13) _____and KAUZAL, G. (1933). PRELIMINARY NOTE ON THE PATHOGENIC IMPORTANCE OF CHABERTIA OVINA (FABRICIUS, 1788). Austral. Vet. Jour. 9: 215-218.

(14) COBBETT, N.G. (1940). AN EFFECTIVE TREATMENT FOR THE CONTROL OF THE SHEEP HEAD GRUB, OESTRUS OVIS, IN AREAS WHERE THE WINTERS ARE COLD. Amer. Vet. Med. Assoc. Jour. 97: 565-570.

(15) DEEM, A.W., and THORP, FRANK, Jr. (1939). VARIATION IN NUMBERS OF COCCIDIA IN LAMBS DURING THE FEEDING SEASON. Vet. Med. 34: 46-47, illus.

(16) Du TOIT, R. (1938). THE EXTERNAL PARASITES OF SHEEP. Farming in South Africa 13: 403-404, 407, illus.

(17) _____and CLARK, R. (1935). THE SHEEP NASAL FLY. A METHOD OF TREATMENT FOR SHEEP INFECTED WITH LARVAE OF OESTRUS OVIS. South African Vet. Med. Assoc. Jour. 6 (1): 25-32, illus.

(18) EDGAR, GRAHAME (1936). FATAL EFFECT OF HEAVY INFESTATION WITH COOPERIA CURTICEI (RAIL LIET, 1893) IN GOATS. Austral. Vet. Jour. 12 (2): 58-61.

(19) FAUST, ERNEST CARROLL (1928). STUDIES ON THELAZIA CALLIPAEDA RAILLIET AND HENRY, 1910. Jour. Parasitol. 15: [75]-86.

(20) FREEBORN, STANLEY B., and BERRY, LESTER J. (1934). OBSERVATIONS ON THE SHEEP TAPEWORM, MONIEZIA EXPANSA, IN CALIFORNIA. Amer. Vet. Med. Assoc. Jour. 85: 611-616, illus.

(21) GILDOW, E.M., and HICKMAN, C.W. (1931). A NEW TREATMENT FOR OESTRUS OVIS LARVAE IN THE HEAD OF SHEEP. Amer. Vet. Med. Assoc. Jour. 79: 211-216, illus.

(22) HERMS, WILLIAM B. (1923). MEDICAL AND VETERINARY ENTOMOLOGY. Ed. 2, 462 pp. illus. New York.

(23) HOBMAIER, ADELE, and HOBMAIER, MICHAEL (1929). UEBER DIE ENTWICKLUNG DES LUNGENWURMES SYNTHETOCAULUS CAPILLARIS IN NACKT-, WEG- UND SCHNIRKELSCHNECKEN. Munchen. Tierarztl. Wchnschr., 80: [497]-500, illus.

(24) _____and HOBMAIER, MICHAEL (1929). DIE ENTWICKLUNG DES LUNGENWURMES DES SCHAFES, DICTYOCAULUS FILARIA RUD., AUSSERHALB UND INNERHALB DES TIERKQRPERS. Munchen. Tierarztl. Wchnschr. 80: [621]-625, illus.

(25) KAUZAL, G. (1932). NOTE ON THE TREATMENT OF LUNG WORM, DICTYOCAULUS FILARIA (RUD., 1809), INFESTATION OF SHEEP. Austral. Vet. Jour. 8: 25-28.

(26) _____(1933). OBSERVATIONS ON THE BIONOMICS OF DICTYOCAULUS FILARIA, WITH A NOTE ON THE CLINICAL MANIFESTATIONS IN ARTIFICIAL INFECTIONS IN SHEEP. Austral. Vet. Jour. 9: 20-26, illus.

(27) _____(1934). OBSERVATIONS ON THE DEVELOPMENT OF RESISTANCE TO DICTYOCAULUS FILARIA. Austral. Vet. Jour. 10: 100-111, illus.

(28) _____(1936). FURTHER STUDIES ON THE PATHOGENIC IMPORTANCE OF CHABERTIA OVINA. Austral. Vet. Jour. 12: 107-110.

(29) _____(1937). A PRELIMINARY STUDY OF THE PATHOGENIC EFFECT OF NEMATODIRUS SPP. IN SHEEP. Austral. Vet. Jour. 13: 120-123.

(30) KEMPER, H.E. (1938). FILARIAL DERMATOSIS OF SHEEP. North Amer. Vet. 19 (9): 36-41, illus.

(31) KRULL, WENDELL H. (1939). OBSERVATIONS ON THE DISTRIBUTION AND ECOLOGY OF THE ORIBATID MITES. Wash. Acad. Sci. Jour. 29: 519-528.

(32) LE ROUX, P.L. (1930). A PRELIMINARY COMMUNICATION ON THE LIFE CYCLE OF COTYLOPHORON COTYLOPHORUM AND ITS PATHOGENICITY FOR SHEEP AND CATTLE. Union So. Africa Dept. Agr. Rpt. Dir. Vet. Serv. and Anim. Indus. 16: 243-253, illus.

(33) MARSH, H., and TUNNICLIFF, E.A. (1941). ENTERITIS IN SHEEP CAUSED BY INFECTION WITH THE PROTOZOAN PARASITE GLOBIDIUM GILRUTHI. Amer. Jour. Vet. Res. 2: 174-177, illus.

(34) MITCHELL, W.C and COBBETT, N.G. (1933). FIELD INVESTIGATIONS RELATIVE TO CONTROL OF OESTRUS OVIS. Amer. Vet. Med. Assoc. Jour. 83: 247-254, illus.

(35) MONNIG, H.O. (1938). VETERINARY HELMINTHOLOGY AND ENTOMOLOGY. THE DISEASES OF DOMESTICATED ANIMALS CAUSED BY HELMINTH AND ARTHROPOD PARASITES. Ed. 2, 409 pp. London.

(36) _____(1940). TREATMENT AGAINST LUNGWORMS (DICTYOCAULUS FILARIA) IN SHEEP. Onderstepoort Jour. Vet. Sci. and Anim. Indus. 14: 111-114.

(37) _____and Du TOIT, R. (1939). THE SHEEP NASAL WORM. Farming in South Africa 14: 242, 251, illus.

(38) NEVEU-LEMAIRE, M. (1936). TRAITE D'HELMINTHOLOGIE MEDICALE ET VETERINAIRE. 1514 pp., illus. Paris.

(39) ORTLEPP, R.J. (1937). OBSERVATIONS ON THE MORPHOLOGY AND LIFE-HISTORY OF GAIGERIA PACHYS CELLS RAILL. AND HENRY, 1910: A HOOKWORM PARASITE OF SHEEP AND GOATS. Onderstepoort Jour. Vet. Sci. and Anim. Indus. 8: 183-212, illus.

(40) _____(1939). OBSERVATIONS ON THE LIFE-HISTORY OF BUNOSTOMUM TRIGONOCEPHALUM, A HOOKWORM OF SHEEP AND GOATS. Onderstepoort Jour. Vet. Sci. and Anim. Indus. 12: 305-318, illus.

(41) RANSOM, B.H. (1913). CYSTICERCUS OVIS, THE CAUSE OF TAPEWORM CYSTS IN MUTTON. Jour. Agr. Res. 1: 15-58, illus.

(42) SHAW, J.N., and SIMMS, B.T. (1930). STUDIES IN FASCIOLIASIS IN OREGON SHEEP AND GOATS. Oreg. Agr. Expt. Sta. Bul. 266, 24 pp., illus.

(43) SHORB, D.A. (1939). PRELIMINARY OBSERVATIONS ON THE EFFECT ON SHEEP OF PURE INFESTATION WITH THE TAPEWORM, MONIEZIA EXPANSA. Helminthol. Soc. Wash. Proc. 6: 77-79, illus.

(44) _____(1940). A NOTE ON THE EFFECT OF TAPEWORM INFESTATION ON THE CONDITION OF SHEEP. Vet. Med. 35: 180-181, illus.

(45) STEWART, J.R. (1932). TREATMENT FOR OESTRUS OVIS. Amer. Vet. Med. Assoc. Jour. 80: 108.

(46) STEWART, M.A. (1940). OVINE THELAZIASIS. Amer. Vet. Med. Assoc. Jour. 96: 486-489.

(47) STUNKARD, HORACE W. (1938). THE DEVELOPMENT OF MONIEZIA EXPANSA IN THE INTERMEDIATE HOST. Parasitology 30: 491-501, illus.

(48) SWALES, W.E. (1935). THE LIFE CYCLE OF FASCIOLOIDES MAGNA (BASSI, 1875), THE LARGE LIVER FLUKE OF RUMINANTS, IN CANADA, WITH OBSERVATIONS ON THE BIONOMICS OF THE LARVAL STAGES AND THE INTERMEDIATE HOSTS, PATHOLOGY OF FASCIOLOIDIASIS MAGNA, AND CONTROL MEASURES. Canad. Jour. Res. 12: 177-215, illus.

(49) SWALES, W.E. (1936). FURTHER STUDIES ON FASCIOLOIDES MAGNA (BASSI, 1875), WARD, 1917, AS A PARASITE OF RUMINANTS. Canad. Jour. Res. Sect. D, Zool. Sci. 14: [83]-95, illus.

(50) THORP, FRANK, Jr. (1938). SOME FEEDLOT DISEASES OF LAMBS. Vet. Med. 33(10): 442-444, illus.

(51) THRELKELD, W.L., and DOWNING, T.O. (1936). A REPORT ON EXPERIMENTAL INFECTIONS OF OVIS ARIES WITH THE INFECTIVE LARVAE OF OSTERTAGIA CIRCUMCINCTA. Jour. Parasitol. 22: [187]-201, illus.

(52) VEGLIA, FRANK (1915). THE ANATOMY AND LIFE-HISTORY OF HAEMONCHUS CONTORTUS (RUD.). Union So. Africa Dept. Agr. Rpts. Dir. Vet. Res. 3 and 4: [347]-500, illus.

(53) _____(1924). PRELIMINARY NOTES ON THE LIFE-HISTORY OF OESOPHAGOSTOMUM COLUMBIANUM. Union So. Africa Dept. Agr. Rpts. Dir. Vet. Ed. and Res. 9 and 10 (1923): [811]-823, illus.

(54) _____(1928). OESOPHAGOSTOMIASIS IN SHEEP (PRELIMINARY NOTE). Dept. Agr. Rpts. Dir. Vet. Ed. and Res. 13 and 14: [755]-797, illus.

(55) WENYON, C.M. (1926). PROTOZOOLOGY. A MANUAL FOR MEDICAL MEN, VETERINARIANS AND ZOOLOGIST. 2 v., 1563 pp., illus. London.

Chapter 5

SHEEP SCAB AND ITS CONTROL

A.W. Miller[1]

[1] *A.W. Miller is Chief, Interstate Inspection Division, Bureau of Animal Industry.*

Scab, which affects the skin and is caused by mange mites, can be had enough on any animal. It is especially serious in the case of sheep because it directly damages the wool; hence the strict Federal quarantines long ago clamped on infected areas. These, and official dipping operations, have been very effective, and sheep scab is now mostly found in farming, not range, areas. Here is what you should do if scab occurs in your flock.

Sheep scab, or scabies, has been known for many centuries; in fact, it is referred to in Leviticus 22: 22, which forbids the use of scabbed sheep in sacrifices.

A half century ago the disease was the greatest draw-back to the sheep industry in the Western States, and it caused heavy losses to feeders in the Corn Belt States also. In fact, sheep scabies was so widespread as to deter many ranchers from engaging in the sheep business, and farmers refused to buy undipped range sheep for feeding purposes. So prevalent was the disease that in 1896 England prohibited the importation of live sheep from the United States.

The parasitic mites that cause scab in sheep are of four species–psoroptic, sarcoptic, chorioptic, and demodectic. Each kind of mite has distinctive habits, with the result that the nature and location of the lesions, or tissue injuries, are more or less characteristic. The psoroptic mites live on the surface of the skin, usually on the withers, back, sides, and rump. The sarcoptic mites burrow into the skin, usually on the head and face or other parts where there is little or no wool. The chorioptic mites live on the surface of the skin, and the lesions they cause are usually found on the legs. The demodectic mites, the smallest in the group, are found in the hair follicles and the glands of the skin, where they cause pimples or nodules.

Psoroptic, Common, or Body Scab

The form of sheep scabies of the greatest economic importance to the sheep industry in the United States is the psoroptic, or common, scab. A highly contagious skin disease readily transmitted from sheep to sheep, it usually spreads rapidly after it is introduced into a flock. The irritation and other effects of the disease make the animals unthrifty and cause loss of weight, a decrease in wool production, and in some instances the death of a large number of affected animals, especially where weather conditions are severe and adequate feed is not available. This form of the disease, however, is rather easily cured by appropriate treatment.

The mites (*Psoroptes equi* var. *ovis*) that cause common scab are white or yellowish and visible to the unaided eye (Fig. 1, *A* & *B*). Their entire life cycle is passed on the body of the host. Each female may deposit 15 to 24 eggs, which usually hatch after 4 to 7 days' incubation. The young mites reach maturity and mate, and females deposit eggs within 10 to 12 days after hatching. These stages in the life history have an important bearing on the interval which should elapse between treatments.

The mites of common, or body, scab prick the skin of the animal to obtain food and probably introduce a poisonous saliva into the wound by this action. As the mites multiply and more wounds are made in the skin, there is itching, inflammation, and exudation of serum. This serum, mixed with particles of dirt and other material, soon hardens and forms scabs. At first only a small pimple can be seen, but as the mites multiply they seek the healthier parts around the edges of the diseased area, and the lesion becomes larger. The affected areas of the skin become hardened and thickened, as may be observed by pinching up a portion and comparing it with the

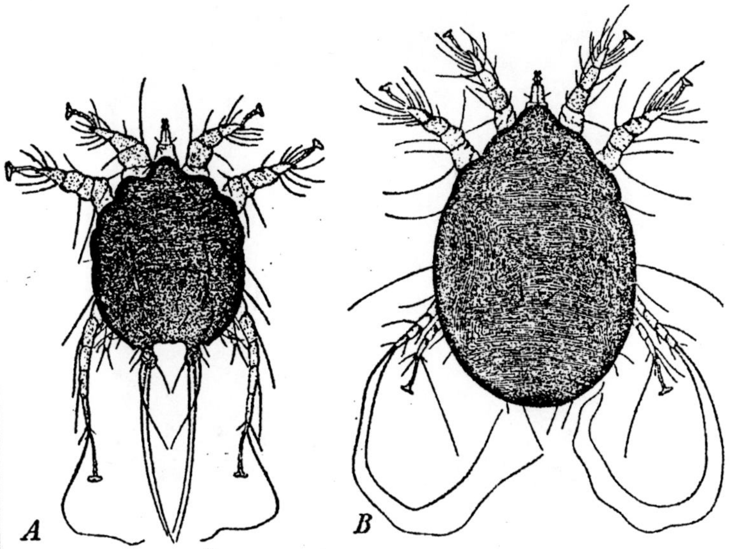

Fig. 1: The psoroptic mites that cause common sheep scab, viewed from above: *A*: Male; *B*: female. Greatly enlarged.

surrounding healthy skin. Infected sheep become restless, scratch themselves, and rub against fences and other members of the flock. The itching becomes more intense when the sheep are warm.

The wool is disturbed; at first slender tags come loose, then the fleece becomes matted, and the sheep pulls out pieces with its mouth. As the disease progresses larger areas become denuded (Fig. 2) until in the advanced stages the skin becomes parchmentlike and greatly thickened and furrowed, and in some instances bleeding occurs in the cracks.

Diagnosis

A definite diagnosis can be made only by demonstrating the presence of the mite that causes common sheep scab. In some instances it is possible to detect the mite in the wool or on the skin of the animal, but the best method is to take scrapings from a recently infected area. When the mites are producing active irritation the surface of the skin in the immediate vicinity of the lesion is greasy

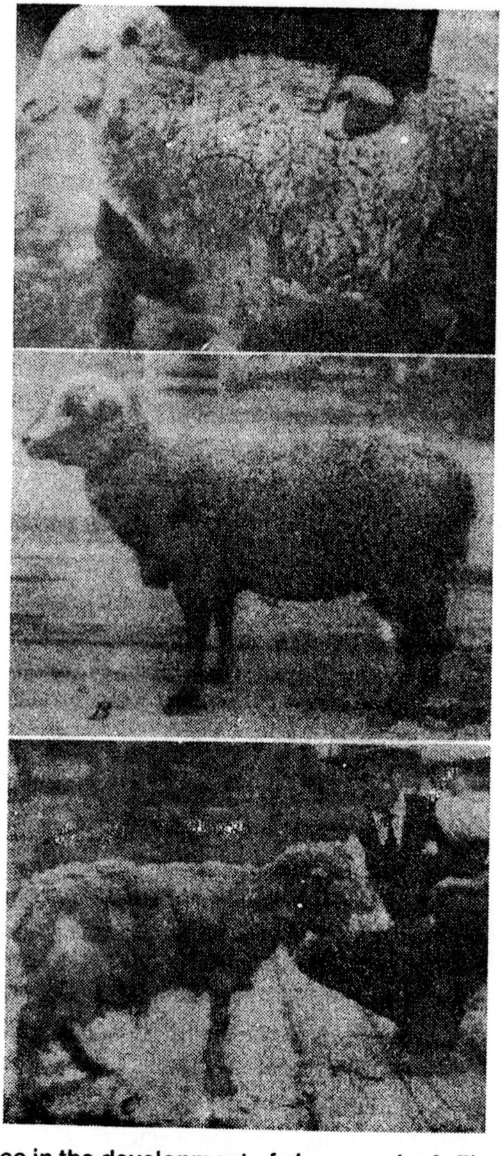

Fig. 2: Stages in the development of sheep scab. *A*: First stage of scab, showing the wool on the shoulder disturbed by biting and scratching; *B*: first break in the fleece; *C*: an advanced case of sheep scab.

and appears bright and glistening or white and glossy. If the lesion is dull and dry it indicates that the mites are inactive at that point and that they will be difficult to find. This condition is usually found in the center of a scabby patch of comparatively long standing. The white glossy appearance is soon in areas of recent infestation or on the outer edges of old lesions, where mites are usually present in large numbers. Scrapings should be taken from such areas.

When the weather is cold the mites are not very active and are difficult to see. If the material taken from an infected area is warmed to about the temperature of the body and placed on a dark background, the mites become more active and can be more readily seen as they move about. A low-power hand lens is a great aid in demonstrating the presence of the mites.

Transmissibility

As already noted, common sheep scab is exceedingly contagious among sheep, but it is not transmissible to other animals except goats. Infected sheep are practically the only source from which sheep scab spreads. Experiments show that clean sheep seldom contract scab from so-called infectious premises. As a precautionary measure, however, such premises should not be used for clean sheep for 30 days after they have been occupied by scabby sheep. Freshly dipped sheep do not become infected from infectious premises, and flocks may safely be held on such premises between the first and second dippings. It is a good sanitary practice, however, to avoid old bed grounds, and small enclosures that have been occupied by scabby sheep should be thoroughly cleaned and disinfected. Sheep scab is transmissible at any season of the year, though during hot, dry weather it often remains dormant, seeming to have been cured. With the advent of cold, rainy weather, however, it again manifests itself.

Treatment

Contrary to the previous opinion that internal medication with sulfur or other medicinal agents would cure the disease, the only effective treatment for common scab is the external application of some medicinal agent that will kill the scab mites. This is best accomplished by dipping, but when dipping is impracticable because of cold weather or for any other reason, isolation of the visibly affected animals and hand dressing of the scabs are advisable. Hand dressing consists in soaking the affected parts with warm dip. In dipping flocks in which the disease is in the advanced stage, animals with hard scabs should be separated from the others just prior to dipping, the scabs soaked with warm dip, and the crusts broken up by rubbing with a stiff brush or stick.

Two dippings are necessary to cure common scab. The first dipping kills the mites but does not destroy all the eggs. The unkilled eggs hatch and form a new generation of mites, which must be destroyed by a second dipping before they have had time to lay eggs. The proper interval between the first and second dippings is 10 to 12 days, but in an emergency it may be extended to a maximum of 14 days.

Many medicinal agents have been used for dips. Some have been found to be useless; others have given satisfactory results in some instances but at other times failed to effect a cure. Workers engaged in sheep scabies eradication realized that a method must be found that would make it possible to maintain dips at a uniform strength throughout the entire dipping operation. After years of experimentation, tests for keeping lime-and-sulfur and nicotine dips uniform were developed. Under existing regulations of the Department of Agriculture, no dip can be used in official dipping of sheep for scabies unless the strength of the bath prepared from it can be satisfactorily determined in the field by a practical, portable testing outfit and unless dipping in a bath of definite strength under actual field conditions will effectually eradicate scabies infection without injury to the animals.

The only dips now permitted in official dipping are those made from lime-sulfur or nicotine. The liquid should be used at a temperature of 95° to 105° F. and must at all times be maintained at a strength of not less than 2 percent of "sulfide sulfur," if it is a lime-sulfur dip, and at not less than 0.05 percent of nicotine, if it is a nicotine dip.

Sarcoptic, or Head, Scab

Sarcoptic scab is not common in the United States. It is difficult to eradicate, but it can be cured. Thorough soaking of the affected parts with warm lime-and-sulfur dip every 5 or 6 days for a month or 6 weeks will usually be effective.

Chorioptic, or Foot, Scab

The form of sheep scabies commonly known as foot scab is caused by a mite (*Chorioptes bovis* var. *ovis*) that closely resembles the psoroptic mite of common sheep scab. The visible lesions usually occur first around the feet but in severe cases may spread to the legs, thighs, and udder, and they are most pronounced during cold weather. The disease is distinguished from common scab by the location of the lesions. This form of sheep scab can be effectively combated with the treatment recommended for common scab. During very cold weather, wading tanks filled with dip may be used instead of dipping vats.

Demodectic, or Follicular, Scab

Demodectic scab is not common in sheep in the United States, but cases have been reported in milk goats. The mite (*Demodex canis* var. *ovis*) that causes this form of scab is not visible to the unaided eye. It is wormlike in form and infests the hair follicles and the sebaceous glands, which lubricate the skin. When present in large numbers the mites cause swellings or nodules that extend deeply into the skin.

No effective method is known for the treatment of flocks infected with demodectic mange. Individual animals that are affected should be removed from the flock and treated or destroyed. Treatment consists in opening all the nodules, removing the contents, and syringing the pockets out with a 2-percent solution of coal-tar-creosote dip.

Dipping Sheep

The method universally practiced in the United States to combat sheep scab is to dip infected and exposed flocks. As already noted, two or more dippings are necessary to effect a cure. All the sheep in a flock should be dipped regardless of the number infected.

In dipping sheep it is most important that close attention be given to numerous details. Sheep should not be dipped immediately after shearing, and great care should be exercised not to dip in a lime-and-sulfur solution any sheep that have unhealed wounds from shear cuts or other causes. Animals with such wounds when dipped in this kind of solution usually develop blood poisoning, the mortality from which is very high. Every possible effort should be made to handle the sheep quietly and to avoid rough treatment of any kind.

Ewes and lambs should be dipped separately as there is great danger of drowning the younger animals if they are dipped together. As ewes recognize their lambs by smell and not by sight, the two groups should be turned together after dipping in order that each mother may have an opportunity to find her lamb.

Several hours before the sheep are to be dipped they should be given a moderate amount of feed and water, but care should be taken to see that they are not too full when dipped. As far as possible, dipping operations should not be undertaken on days when the weather is extremely cold and stormy. If it is necessary in an emergency to dip sheep during winter weather, the operation should be completed early in the day in order that the animals may have time to dry off and be fed before night.

The quantity of dip in the vat should be sufficient to submerge the sheep completely, and the liquid should be maintained at a temperature of 95° to 105° F. An accurate thermometer should be provided and the temperature checked frequently. The sheep should be kept in the dipping vat long enough for the wool to become fairly well saturated; in the case of infected sheep this will not be less than 2 minutes. In well-advanced cases the hard scabs should be broken up and soaked with the dipping fluid, but in dressing such areas care should be taken not to cause the wounds to bleed, as the blood may protect the mites from the effects of the dip.

While being put in the vat, the animals should be carefully watched by men with dipping forks stationed along the file of sheep to see that the dipping is properly done and to prevent accidents (Fig. 3). As soon as the dip becomes dirty it should be changed regardless of the number of sheep that have been dipped in it. When lime-and-sulfur dip is used, the solution should be changed after it is 10 days old. Only dips permitted by the Department of Agriculture should be used in the treatment of sheep against scabies. As already noted, it is essential that the dip be maintained at the required strength at all times. By frequent testing of the solution with the field tests available for lime-and-sulfur and nicotine dips it is possible to determine when it is necessary to add fresh dip to maintain the required strength.

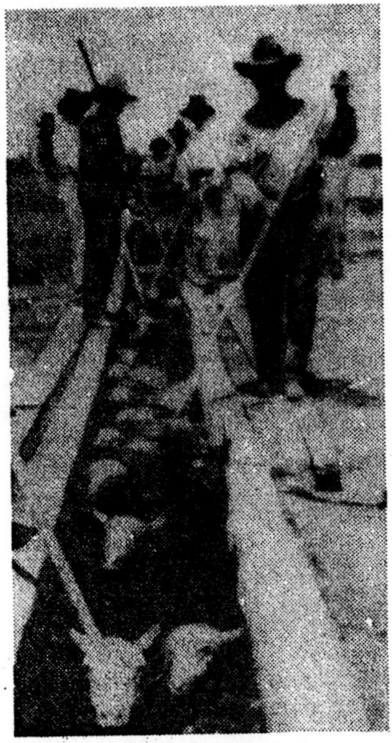

Fig. 3: Dipping sheep to control scab. The dipping forks (poles with hooks) are used to control the movement of sheep through the dipping vat and also to force their heads under the surface momentarily to make sure that all the scab mites are reached by the dip.

Conduct of Control Work

In June 1897 the Department of Agriculture issued an order governing the transportation of sheep affected with scabies, and Federal inspectors were placed at the principal feeding points of all the railroads leading to market centers to inspect and supervise the shipping of sheep. In 1899 an order was issued requiring that all sheep shipped from stockyards to other States for feeding purposes be dipped, and in July of that year another order forbade any sheep affected with scabies to be shipped interstate that had not been dipped in a mixture approved by the Department.

The following year inspectors were stationed at a number of points in the Western range States, and various livestock sanitary officials issued dipping orders. This plan was more satisfactory to the sheep growers and transportation companies than the previous one, but still the desired results were not accomplished. Accordingly, on June 1, 1905, a Federal quarantine was placed on all the territory west of the eastern border of North Dakota, South Dakota, Kansas, Oklahoma, and Texas, an area of more than 1,700,000 square miles.

Under cooperative arrangements with the livestock sanitary officials of the several states, systematic inspections by State and Federal employees were made of all sheep in infected localities, and all flocks found to be infected or exposed were dipped under official supervision. This work was supplemented by rigid inspection of sheep arriving at public stockyards and appropriate treatment or other disposition of those classed as infected or exposed. When this work was inaugurated 90 percent of all the bands of sheep in some States were infected with scabies. Progress toward the eradication of the disease continued, and from time to time the quarantine on various areas was lifted. At the present time only small areas in two States are under Federal quarantine for this disease. So successful has the eradication work been that most of the range States in which the sheep industry is important have been entirely free from the disease for several years. The remaining infection is largely confined to a few farming States where numerous auction markets and the almost exclusive use of trucks for transportation have made the eradication problem a difficult one.

Control work is conducted at present under cooperative agreement between the United States Bureau of Animal Industry and the livestock sanitary officials of the various States. The agreements specify in some detail the part that each of these cooperative agencies shall take in the work of eradication. Generally both parties to an agreement furnish trained men to make inspections and supervise the dipping of infected and exposed flocks.

In recent years the States with few exceptions have handled the quarantine of flocks and areas infected with sheep scab so effectively that it has not been necessary to impose Federal quarantines. The situation in several of the farming States has been rather serious during recent years, however. The indiscriminate movement of sheep through auction markets in these States and their uncontrolled transportation by trucks have presented a difficult problem, but it is being gradually solved by the enforcement of State regulations at the auction markets and by the active cooperation of Federal and State inspectors in locating centers of infection and enforcing appropriate control measures when diseased flocks are found.

Flock owners who plan to dip sheep of their own accord are strongly advised to have the work supervised by a veterinarian or other properly trained and equipped person who is experienced in dealing with sheep scab and prepared to test the strength of the dip. Flock owners are reminded also that for their own protection and that of the community they should report the appearance of sheep scab promptly to the nearest veterinarian, State livestock official, or representative of the Bureau of Animal Industry. These professional workers are prepared to take suitable action to eradicate the infection.

Chapter 6

SHEEP TICKS

Marion Imes & O.G. Babcock[1]

[1] *Marion Imes is Senior Veterinarian, Zoological Division, Bureau of Animal Industry, and O.G. Babcock is Associate Entomologist, Division of Insects Affecting Man and Animals, Bureau of Entomology and Plant Quarantine.*

The sheep tick, which is not a tick at all but a fly, can do a good deal of damage to fleeces, besides causing a serious set-back in lambs. A number of substances, used as dips according to the directions in this article, will control these parasites.

The sheep tick or ked (*Melophagus ovinus*) is not a true tick but a wingless parasitic fly that lives in the fleece of sheep. The adult female is about one-quarter of an inch long and the male is slightly smaller (Fig. 1, *A* & *B*). The ticks are brown, have six legs, and are plainly visible to the unaided eye.

Sheep ticks are widely distributed, occurring in practically all parts of the United States where sheep are kept, and affecting primarily the coarse-wool and medium-wool breeds, and sometimes Angora goats. The fine-wool breeds of sheep are usually not affected to any great extent; the parasites apparently are not adapted to thrive in their tight, greasy fleeces.

In obtaining their food, sheep ticks puncture the skin and suck blood and lymph from the host animal. They do not remain attached in one place like true ticks but move about in the fleece, making a new puncture each time they feed. Hence when sheep are grossly

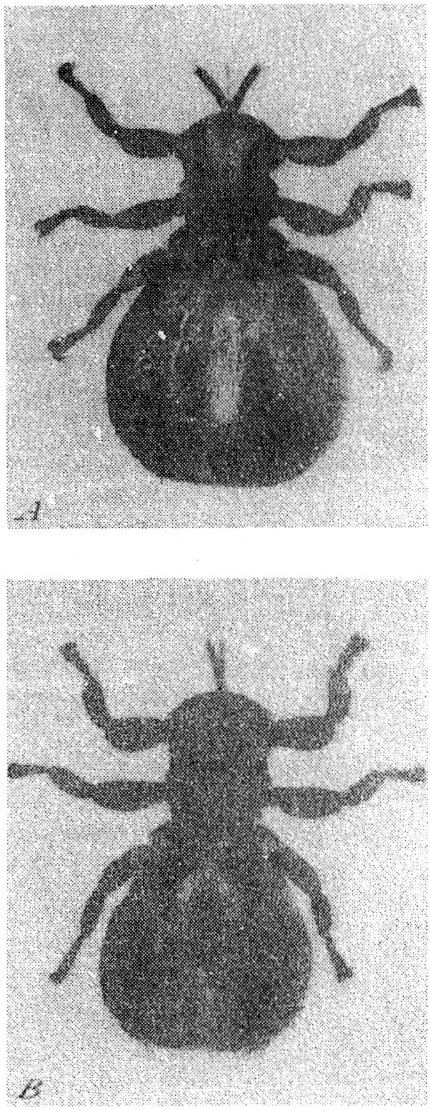

Fig. 1: *A*: An engorged female sheep tick, under side (× 10),
B: A mature sheep tick, upper side (× 10).

infested many punctures are made in the skin, and the resulting intense itching and irritation cause the animals to become restless so that they do not eat well or gain weight normally. To relieve the itching, infested sheep rub, bite, and scratch themselves, with the result that the fleeces are disarranged, tufts of wool are pulled out, and some of the wool fibers are broken or damaged. Since losses in body weight and damage to fleeces reduce the value of sheep, it is profitable to the flock owner to control or eradicate sheep ticks.

Life History

The four stages in the life cycle of the sheep tick are the egg, the larva, the pupa, and the adult or sexually mature parasite. The egg is not laid but is retained in the body of the female, where it develops into a larva in about 7 days. At the time of birth the larva is covered with a soft white membrane, which turns brown and becomes a hard shell or puparium in about 12 hours (Fig. 2). The puparium is attached to the wool fibers of the sheep by a gluelike substance that is soluble in water.

The pupal stage of the insect is passed in the shell, or puparium. These shell-covered pupae are commonly called eggs. In 19 to 24 days from the time it is deposited, the shell of the pupa is broken

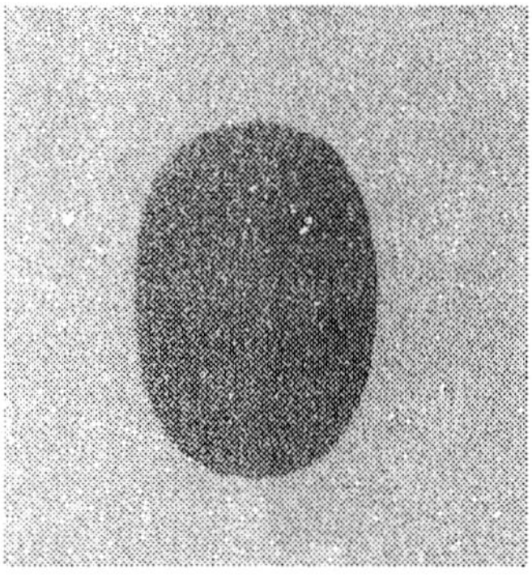

Fig. 2: Sheep tick pupa (× 10). Pupae are attached to the wool fibers; because of their hard shells they are commonly called eggs.

open at one end and the young tick emerges to become active in the fleece. The duration of the pupal stage, usually called the period of incubation, is influenced by the weather. During warm weather the average period of incubation on the host is about 19 days, while during cold weather it is 24 days of longer.

After emerging from the puparium the young tick develops rapidly and reaches sexual maturity in 3 or 4 days. The female usually deposits it first pupa within 8 to 10 days after mating. From the practical standpoint the two important stages in the life cycle may be summarized as follows: When about 14 days old the female tick deposits its first pupa; from this pupa a young tick emerges in about 19 to 24 days.

Habits and Spread

Each female sheep tick produces an average of 12 to 15 pupae during its lifetime, one being deposited about every 7 or 8 days. The pupae are attached to the wool fibers from ½ to 1 inch from the skin. Thus when the sheep are shorn the majority of the pupae and some of the ticks are removed with the fleece. As freshly shorn sheep offer little protection for the ticks, they usually migrate in large numbers to the unshorn lambs during the shearing season. When lambs become heavily infested they receive a setback at an important period in their development, which causes considerable financial loss to the owner.

When separated from their host, adult sheep ticks live only about 4 days. Dislodged pupae, however, may retain their vitality during warm weather and emerge as active young ticks in due time, when they attach themselves to sheep at the first opportunity. Pupae dislodged from sheep during cold weather do not complete their development, as freezing temperatures kill them.

It is evident that premises occupied by ticky sheep may become infested, especially during warm weather. A safe basis of practice is to consider that buildings, corrals, and pastures occupied by tick sheep remain infested during warm weather for about 60 days after the sheep are removed. Before infested stables, corrals, or other small enclosures are used for clean sheep, the premises should be cleaned and disinfected. All litter should be removed down to a smooth surface, then all exposed surfaces sprayed with coal-tar creosote diluted in accordance with the directions on the container. As the disinfectant probably will not destroy the vitality of the pupae, cleaning should be done thoroughly so that pupae will be removed with the litter, which should be plowed under, burned, or otherwise destroyed. Since it is not practical to clean and disinfect large areas, infected pastures should not be used for clean sheep during warm weather. About 2 months after all infested sheep have been removed, pastures may be considered safe for use.

When sheep ticks are introduced into a flock they spread rapidly. Among farm sheep this occurs especially during cold weather when the sheep usually come in close contact with one another, but it occurs at all seasons among range sheep which are usually closely herded, crowded into corrals, and in close contact on the bed grounds.

Detecting Ticks on Sheep

When sheep are heavily infested with sheep ticks they bite and scratch themselves and rub against any available object, including other members of the flock. These efforts to relieve the intense itching caused by the ticks disturb and damage the wool, giving the fleece a ragged appearance.

Sheep ticks may sometimes be seen crawling over the tips of the wool fibers during warm weather, but usually they remain deep in the fleece, especially during cold weather. Their favourite locations on the animal are the neck, breast, shoulders, belly, and thighs, where the fleece is thin and the skin tender. In examining sheep for ticks the wool over these regions should be parted. If ticks are present, they and the pupae can be easily seen.

The first symptoms of tick infestation are similar to those of scabies, lice, wildfire, and other conditions that cause intense itching. Finding ticks on sheep, therefore, does not exclude other possible causes of itching and irritation, and the examination should be thorough to assure that other causes have not been overlooked.

Eradication or Control by Dipping

The only known practical method of eradicating sheep ticks is to dip the infested sheep in a liquid that will kill the parasites. Killing the adult ticks by dipping is a simple matter, but the pupae, which are more resistant to dips, may complete their development and produce a new crop of ticks. To complete the eradication it is necessary to kill the newly hatched ticks before they are old enough to deposit pupae. This may be done either by dipping the sheep again after an interval of 24 to 28 days or by using a dip that will remain active in the fleece long enough to destroy the young ticks after they emerge from the shell.

Fall dipping is good insurance against the ravages of ticks during the winter when the weather is too cold for dipping. If the lambs become heavily infested shortly after shearing, which often occurs, the flock should be dipped as soon as the shear cuts heal.

In dipping sheep for ticks, the depth of the dip in the vat should be 40 to 48 inches or deep enough to swim the tallest animal.[2] All members of the flock, regardless of the number showing infestation, should be dipped, as well as all animals of other species running with the flock. The animals should be held in the dip about 1 minute, or long enough to saturate the fleece. The head of each animal should be submerged, or ducked, twice for an instant. It is not necessary to heat dips used for sheep ticks, but the temperature of the liquid should not be low enough to chill the animals.

The three kinds of dips commonly used when sheep are dipped twice for sheep ticks are nicotine, coal-tar creosote, and cresol. These dips are concentrated liquids sold under various trade names, and directions for diluting and using them are supplied with each package or container. They are effective in eradicating sheep ticks when used in fairly soft water.

There are also three classes or kinds of dips used for eradicating sheep ticks at one dipping, namely, fused-bentonite-sulfur-cube, arsenic-sulfur-rotenone, and home-made derris or cube dip. The first two are proprietary products sold under different trade names. When used according to the instructions furnished by the manufacturers with each package, they are effective in eradicating sheep ticks. In using products containing arsenic it should be remembered that it is a poison, and proper precaution should be taken to avoid injury to men and animals.

Derris powder, the pulverized roots of a shrub that grows in the Tropics of the Old World, and cube powder, made from the roots of

---

[2] IMES, MARION. THE SHEEP TICK AND ITS ERADICATION BY DIPPING. U.S. Dept. Agr. Farmers' Bul. 798, 22 pp., illus. 1917. (Revised, 1932 and 1940).

plants found in South America, are among the effective insecticides that have come into general use during recent years. One of the active ingredients of both these powders is rotenone, and they are about equally effective as remedies for external parasites of animals. Powders commercially classed as containing 5 percent of rotenone are generally used.

In making home-made derris or cube dip, either derris powder or cube powder may be used. To prepare derris or cube dip fill the dipping vat with water to the dip line and add the powder in the proportion of 1 pound to each 100 gallons of water. Mix the powder with a small quantity of water to form a thin paste and distribute it over the surface of the water in the vat. When the contents of the vat are well stirred so the paste is uniformly mixed with the water, the dip is ready for use. Freshly prepared dip should always be used, since old dip which has stood in the vat for several days is no longer suitable.

Chapter 7

GOAT LICE

O.G. Babcock & Emory C. Cushing[1]

[1] *O.G. Babcock is Associate Entomologist and Emory C. Cushing is Senior Entomologist, Division of Insects Affecting Man and Animals, Bureau of Entomology and Plant Quarantine.*

Two kinds of blue lice, two kinds of red lice, and a large yellow louse attack goats. Although they are the worst external parasite the goat keeper has to contend with, he can get rid of them with very little trouble if he will follow the directions given here.

Lice are the most widespread and probably the most important external parasites of goats of all breeds in the United States. Yet the control of these pests is not difficult, and there would seem to be little reason for goat raisers throughout the country to sustain the losses that are at present caused by these parasites year after year.

Species, Life History, and Spread of Goat Lice

Goats are commonly infested with five species of lice, two of which (*Linognathus stenopsis* and *L. africanus*), called blue lice, feed by puncturing the skin and sucking blood. The other three have mouth parts fitted for chewing and feed on the hair, scales from the skin, and extraneous matter on the skin surface. Of these three species, one (*Bovicola penicillata*) is commonly referred to as the large yellow or hairy louse and the other two (*B. limbatus* and *B. caprae*) as red lice.

The different species of goat lice have much the same breeding habits, and their life cycles are similar. Ordinarily, goat lice spend their entire lives on the bodies of goats; they mate, lay their eggs, and develop without leaving the host. Sometimes other animals such as sheep, dogs, and burros that are in close association with infested flocks may act as temporary carriers of goat lice, but they are not subject to true infestations.

The nits, or eggs of the lice, are laid in the fleece and are attached firmly to the hair close to the skin. Quite often an egg is cemented to more than one fiber, which accounts for the matting of the hair frequently seen in heavily infested animals. The eggs hatch in 7 to 14 days, depending on the temperature of the air.

After hatching, the immature louse must shed its skin twice before reaching the adult stage. The first molt occurs 2 to 10 days after hatching and the second 3 to 13 days after the first. As many as 15 days after the second molt are sometimes required for the young lice to become sexually mature. The entire life cycle of goat lice from the time the eggs are laid until full maturity is reached ranges in length from 14 to 75 days.

Infestations of goat lice are easily detected, although newly hatched lice are almost transparent and it is difficult to see them. The adults can readily be seen with the unaided eye, however, and the fact that in ordinary infestations all stages are present on the goat at the same time makes detection easy. During the summer months the number of lice on the animals is greatly reduced, but it increases rapidly through the fall and winter.

Lice do not remain attached in one place as do true ticks but move about over the body of the animal, feeding at frequent intervals and causing a constant and extreme itching and irritation of the skin.

Because of the annoyance occasioned by both sucking and biting lice, the infested animals are restless and do not feed well; hence they lose weight, become unthrifty, and show signs of low vitality (Fig. 1) . The mohair becomes ragged and broken from scratching, biting, and rubbing. The fibers are weakened, lack luster, and become matted, tangled, and discoluored. In some sections of the country where goat raising and mohair production have been highly developed, ranchmen recognize that in heavily infested flocks the

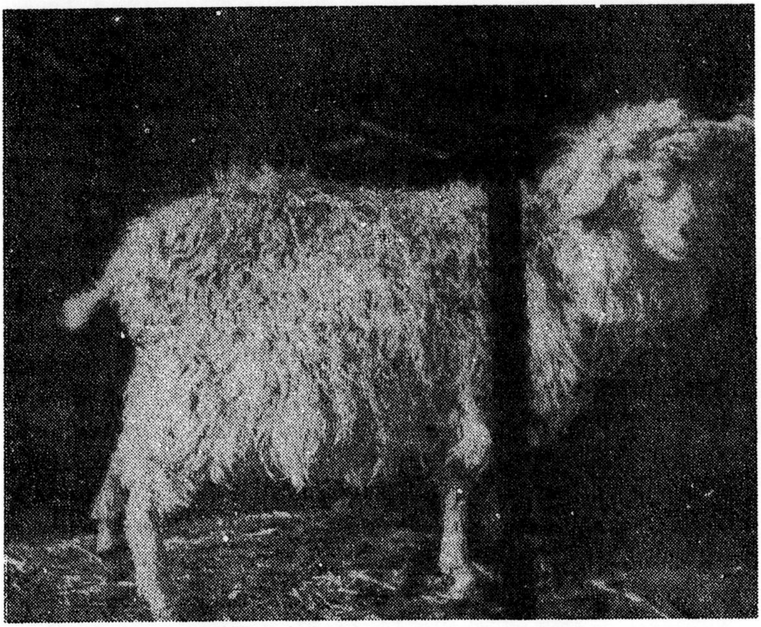

Fig. 1: Goat heavily infested with lice.

quality and quantity of mohair are greatly reduced, the actual loss amounting to as much as one-half pound of mohair per animal. Moreover, infested animals are apt to scratch themselves on sharp objects, such as pointed broken boards, protruding nails in corrals, and wire fences, with the result that the skin is often broken, making wounds that are susceptible to screwworm infestation, which may cause further losses.

Kids and the old, weak, unthrifty animals of the flock are usually the most heavily infested.

When introduced into a clean herd, goat lice spread rapidly from one animal to another, especially during cold weather or when the animals are confined in close contact with one another. The spread of the infestation is due chiefly to the direct contact of lousy animals with uninfested ones. It is possible, however, for an infestation to start among clean goats that are confined on premises previously occupied by lousy animals, owing to the fact that under favourable conditions some adult lice may live apart from a host for periods of 3 to 18 days, particularly in warm weather. The nits attached to dislodged hair may continue to hatch for several days, and the young lice may live for 3 or 4 days.

Control and Eradication

Goat lice are probably more easily eliminated, usually at less expense in money and labour, than any other group of insect parasites of domestic animals. Several insecticides that are cheap and readily available are effective in killing these insects.

The blue, or sucking, lice are harder to kill and inflict greater injury than the biting lice, but both can be eradicated by proper control practices.

Perhaps the simplest method, and the only effective one for eradicating the lice, is to dip the goats in a water solution or suspension of the louse-killing material. Since it is not advisable to use this treatment in cold weather, when the lice become much more numerous, the owner should not wait until winter to begin control treatments. When infestations become so heavy during the winter that treatments are imperative, if only a few animals are involved, they may be hand-dusted with an insecticide to keep the parasites in check. Although this cannot be depended upon to kill all the lice, it will greatly reduce their number and prevent severe injury to the goats. Spraying is sometimes resorted to, but, like hand dusting, it is not completely effective.

The best time to dip Angora goats is 1 month to 6 weeks after they are sheared, provided this permits the dipping to be done before cold weather. If Angoras are treated too short a time before shearing, the insecticides may lower the quality of the fleece by removing some of the natural oil. Furthermore, animals dipped when they have a heavy fleece carry out more dip, which increases the cost of the treatment. A month to 6 weeks after shearing, the fleece is heavy enough to retain a sufficient amount of the insecticide to kill the lice, but it does not retain excessive amounts of the dip.

Goats of breeds other than Angora may be treated at any time when weather conditions are favourable.

None of the insecticides now recommended is effective in killing louse eggs, and since these may continue to hatch for 10 or 12 days, it is necessary to follow the first dipping with a second one in 11 to 16 days. Usually two dippings are sufficient to eradicate all the lice in a flock, provided every animal is found and treated. When lice make their appearance in a flock it is always advisable to treat every animal. The dipped animals should then be turned into pastures that have not been occupied by goats for the previous 4 to 6 weeks.

Insecticides for Killing Goat Lice

Several materials are useful for treating goats infested with lice. All of them have certain disadvantages, but they are about equally effective in eradicating the parasites. Finely ground sulfur, 98 percent of which will pass through a sieve having 325 meshes to the inch, is one of the simplest. Since the sulfur particles are not wetted by contact with water, it is necessary to combine the material with a so-called wetting agent, which permits the mixing of the sulfur with water and holds the particles in suspension so that they become enmeshed in the hair of the animal when it is dipped. Commercial companies now supply, at reasonable prices, wettable sulfur-that is, sulfur with a wetting agent added–already prepared, and it is advisable for goat raisers to purchase sulfur in this form rather than attempt to prepare the mixture themselves. All wettable sulfurs do not combine well in hard water, especially those containing relatively large amounts of alkali and gypsum but the use of certain wetting agents will largely overcome this difficulty. Goat raisers in the United States who have not had previous experience with the use of sulfur in their present localities should request the advice of the United States Department of Agriculture regarding the proper material to use.

Wettable sulfur kills lice slowly, requiring from 7 to 10 days to effect a complete kill. It is not known definitely how sulfur kills the lice, but the available evidence indicates that a gas, hydrogen sulfide, is given off as a result of the contact of the sulfur with the animal, and that this gas destroys the insects. In preparation for dippings the sulfur is mixed with water at the rate of 10 pounds per 100 gallons. A mixture of wettable sulfur and one of the powdered insecticidal plant materials, cube or derris, containing at least 4 to 5 percent rotenone is somewhat more efficient in killing lice than sulfur alone. Fifty pounds of wettable sulfur plus 10 pounds of either cube or derris powder per 1,000 gallons of water makes an efficient dip. The same combination in these proportions of sulfur and cube or derris is a good dust for hand treating infested goats; or sulfur cube, or derris may be used alone. An ounce or two per animal is sufficient for one treatment.

Prepared arsenical dips which are available on the market and are recommended by the Government for use in dipping cattle to remove the cattle fever tick are also suitable for the control of goat lice. The instructions on the label of the container should be followed closely in diluting and using ready-prepared arsenical dips. Since they are poisonous to animals when taken internally, care should be taken that the animals do not drink any of the dip. The vat should not be emptied where the liquid will soil pasture or feed, and the freshly treated animals should be held in a drain pen or a suitable inclosure where the dip dripping from them cannot form pools. Men working around the vat should be careful not to get their clothing wet with the arsenical solution, and should wash their hands frequently to prevent possible absorption of the arsenic.

When used with soft water, coal-tar-creosote dips, sold under various trade names, are effective for the control of goat lice. In hard water the ingredients often separate, and injury to the animals and the fleeces results.

Treating Infested Goats

Where only a small number of animals are to be treated, a large washtub or a small galvanized-iron tank will suffice, but when several hundred animals are to be dipped, it is more convenient and economical to construct a special vat. The round vat shown in figure 2 has proved the most economical for the dipping of goats alone. If it is necessary to dip horses, cattle, and other large animals also, it is advisable to construct a rectangular vat. Specifications for these vats may be obtained from the United States Department of Agriculture.

The animals should not be dipped if there is likely to be a cold wave before they become thoroughly dry. Dipping in excessively hot weather also should be avoided. The animals should not be driven any distance just before or very soon after dipping. Care in throwing them into the vat will help to avoid injuries and reduce the possibility of strangling. In fact, quiet, careful handling is essential to get the best results and to prevent losses.

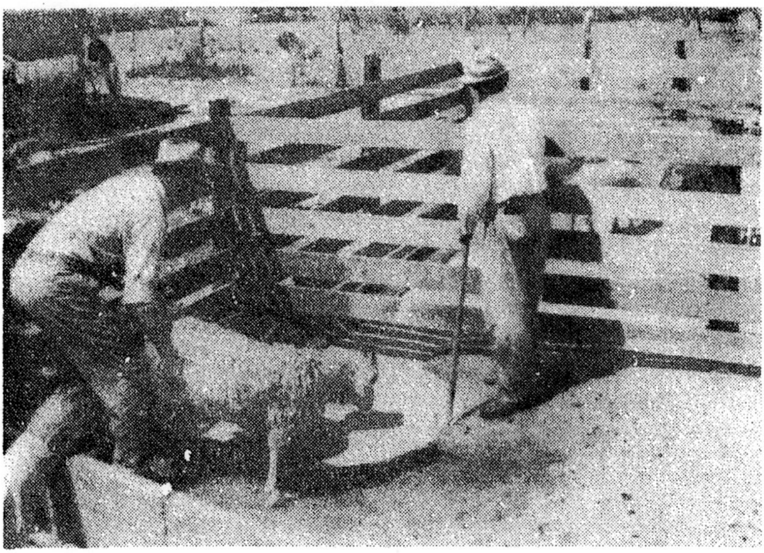

Fig. 2: A round vat for dipping goats.

The animal should be kept in the dip approximately 1 minute. When it comes to the surface after the first immersion, it should be allowed to get its breath, then its head should be ducked beneath the surface momentarily, and it should receive another ducking before leaving the vat.

The dipping fluid in the vat should always be 40 to 60 inches deep. In estimating the amount of dip required to treat a flock, allow at least 2 quarts for each freshly sheared goat and about 1 gallon for each full-fleeced animal.

Further Studies on the Control of Goat Lice

Dips now recommended for the control of goat lice are sometimes toxic to the animals and none of them destroy the eggs. Research is being carried on to find a nonpoisonous insecticide that will kill all lice and eggs in a single application. Such a dip would eliminate much of the time and labour required in using present remedies that must be applied two or three times a season to effect control. Results of recent experiments encourage the belief that such an insecticide will soon be found.

Chapter 8

PREGNANCY DISEASE OF SHEEP

M.S. Shahan[1]

[1] *M.S. Shahan is Veterinarian, Pathological Division, Bureau of Animal Industry.*

Ninety percent of the ewes affected by pregnancy disease die within 1 to 10 days. Although the cause of the disease is not known, it is very probably due to poor nutrition and lack of exercise during pregnancy. Hence it is largely preventable by the methods here suggested.

The unobstructed development of pregnancy disease in a flock or band of pregnant ewes often leads to disastrous losses. Frequently as many as one-fourth of the group develop the disease and 9 of every 10 sick animals die, most of the lambs being lost as well as the mothers.

Although the disease is also known as preparturient paralysis, acidosis of pregnant ewes, lambing paralysis, "pregnancy ketosis", pregnancy toxemia, and old ewe disease, the term "pregnancy disease" is at present generally preferred because of the primary association of the condition with pregnancy and the lack of complete scientific evidence as to its exact character. Apparently its distribution is worldwide, and no part of the United States is free from it so far as is known. The ailment is primarily one of pregnant ewes, especially those carrying twins or triplets, though occasionally those with only one lamb in the uterus are affected. Usually the ewes are in the fourth or the fifth (last) month of pregnancy when the disease occurs.

Ewes from 3 to 6 years old appear to be more commonly affected than younger or older ewes. The condition is more common in small farm flocks than in large bands on the range. There is no generally accepted evidence that one breed is more likely to develop the disease than others, although the breeds or strains that normally produce a considerable proportion of twins and triplets may be more frequently affected, other things being equal, than breeds or strains producing single lambs predominantly.

The ailment has been observed in well-nourished as well as in poorly nourished ewes. Because of ignorance, lack of adequate facilities, or protracted inclement weather, pregnant ewes may be so closely confined that they do not get enough exercise. Often, for the same or other reasons, they are poorly or unwisely fed. Either of these conditions appears to be especially conducive to pregnancy disease.

Cause of Pregnancy Disease

Pregnancy, poor feeding, and lack of exercise appear to be the chief factors causing the disease. No evidence that infection plays a part has been found. Although it has been very difficult for those studying the disease to produce it experimentally, the prevailing opinion is that it is of metabolic origin (*1, 4, 5, 6, 8*)[2], that is, it is associated with the processes by which the animal body transforms feedstuffs into tissue elements and converts complex substances in the feed into simpler ones in the production of energy.

Pregnancy in any case is a critical period for the ewe. In addition to preserving and nourishing her own body, including the fleece, through the feed she consumes, the pregnant ewe is furnishing food for the development of the unborn lamb. If there is more than one fetus, the need for minerals, proteins, carbohydrates, and the other food elements is correspondingly increased.

With the growth and development of the fetus, the tax on the mother increases. The eliminative processes, functioning to rid the body of waste materials, are often greatly impaired in the later stages

---

[2] Italic numbers in parentheses refer to Literature Cited.

of pregnancy. The accumulation of waste products, which may assume the nature of poisons or toxins, seriously affects her well-being, and consequently that of the unborn offspring. In cases of pregnancy disease, a definite acidosis, or reduction in the alkali reserves of the body, develops. This is believed to result primarily from impaired metabolism of carbohydrates and fats.

Before the development of definite, clear-cut, outward symptoms of the disease in affected ewes, primary evidences may be detectable in the blood or urine by analysis in the laboratory. These evidences consist essentially of an increase in the ketone bodies (complex acids derived from fat metabolism) and a decrease in the normal blood sugar. With the progress of the disease, these changes become more marked. The relationships of other factors in pregnancy disease have as yet not been proved.

Symptoms and Post Mortem Findings

The death of one or more ewes in a flock just before lambing time justifies suspicion of pregnancy disease. The first sign of the disease (2, 3, 4) may be the lagging of one or more of the ewes when the flock is being driven. An affected ewe nearly always grinds her teeth, appears dull and weak, urinates frequently, and trembles when exercised. Later, she refuses feed, drinks little water, urinates less and less often, breathes rapidly, becomes stupid or highly nervous, appears to be blind and finally loses the power to stand, going down in a few hours or after 1 or 2 days. Animals affected with pregnancy disease often lie on the sternum (breast) with the head turned around to the side of the body, much like a cow with parturient paresis, or milk fever. They may lie in this position or flat on the side for days. Usually there is no fever. The disease lasts from 1 to 10 days, and death results in more than 90 percent of the cases. If lambing should occur, however, especially during the early stages of the disease, recovery usually follows. The lambs are likely to be weak and usually die, either from the toxic effect of the disease or because the amount of milk given by the ewe is not sufficient to sustain life.

Ewes that die of pregnancy disease almost invariably are carrying more than one fetus in the uterus. Usually the carcass contains little fat, but sometimes there is a normal or even more than normal amount, which frequently has a dull, mottled appearance. The most striking changes observed in post mortem examination are in the liver, which appears to be thickened and is of a light yellowish-brown colour. Microscopically it is found to be affected by severe fatty degeneration, and chemically there is a decrease in glycogen (a form of body sugar). The kidneys also are usually pale and softened.

Prevention and Treatment

The prevention of pregnancy disease, as of most diseases, is much more practical and economical than treatment. Fortunately, enough is known about the disease to prevent in ill most cases. Of first importance is the feeding of proper rations. The principles of good feeding are outlined in A Handbook for Better Feeding of Livestock (*8*), as well as in more detailed form the 1939 Yearbook of Agriculture, Food and Life (*9*). Throughout pregnancy, ewes that are not on good green pasture should receive a liberal allowance of clean, bright legume hay. In addition, especially during the last month or two of pregnancy, they should receive good, sound grain daily, beginning with one-fourth of a pound a day during the eighth to the sixth week before lambing, and the amount should be gradually increased to 1 pound during the fourth to the second weeks. Ewes in good condition may not require more than half a pound daily during the latter period, and very fat ewes may need little or nothing more than good pasture or a liberal supply of legume hay. With the grain ration, small quantities of molasses, pure dextrose, corn sirup, or brown sugar may be given. A constant supply of salt is necessary, and regular hours of feeding are desirable. Abrupt changes in the kind or amount of feed should not be made.

A moderate amount of exercise is essential. Ewes in good condition should have more than those that are weak and thin, but in all cases the animals should be taken some distance, at least a quarter of a mile if possible, from the bedding ground or shed for feeding. If it is impossible to provide exercise in this way because of deep snow or other conditions, some other method should be used. Rapid, forced driving, however, is not desirable, especially for thin ewes.

Treatment of advanced cases of pregnancy disease is rarely successful. Sometimes, however, recovery may be effected by the injection of certain sugar solutions into the blood stream, and such other appropriate treatments may be given as are believed by the veterinarian to be advisable. Certain glandular products have been tried experimentally, but there is not yet conclusive proof of their efficacy. Cases detected in the earliest stages by tests of the blood or urine for ketone bodies may recover if given corn syrup or some other form of dextrose, either on the feed, by stomach tube, or by injection into the blood stream.

Literature Cited

(1) CAMERON, H.S., and GOSS, H. (1940). PREPARTURIENT PARESIS IN EWES. Amer. Vet. Med. Assoc. Jour. 96: 165-169, illus.

(2) ELDER, CECIL, and UREN, A.W. (1940). PREGNANCY DISEASE OF SHEEP. Mo. Agr. Expt. Sta. Bul. 412, 16 pp., illus.

(3) MARSH, HADLEIGH (1929). SOME OBSCURE DISEASES OF SHEEP. Amer. Vet. Med. Assoc. Jour. 74: 724-735.

(4) RODERICK, LEE M., and HARSHFIELD, G.S. (1932). PREGNANCY DISEASE OF SHEEP. N. Dak. Agr. Expt. Sta. Tech. Bul. 261, 31 pp., illus.

(5) _____HARSHFIELD, G.S., and HAWN, M.C. (1937). THE PATHOGENESIS OF KETOSIS: PREGNANCY DISEASE OF SHEEP. Amer. Vet. Med. Assoc. Jour 90: 41-50.

(6) SAMPSON, J., GONZAGA, A.C., and HAYDEN, C.E. (1933). THE KETONES OF THE BLOOD AND URINE OF THE COW AND EWE IN HEALTH AND DISEASE. Cornell Vet. 23: 184-207.

(7) _____and HAYDEN, C.E. (1936). PHYSIOLOGICAL ASPECTS OF KETOSIS IN COWS AND EWES WITH SPECIAL REFERENCE TO CARBOHYDRATE METABOLISM. Cornell Vet. 26: 183-199. illus.

(8) SHEETS, E.W., and JACKSON, WILLIAM, compilers (1924). A HANDBOOK FOR BETTER FEEDING OF LIVESTOCK. U.S. Dept. Agr. Misc. Cir. 12, 48 pp.

(9) UNITED STATES DEPARTMENT OF AGRICULTURE (1939). FOOD AND LIFE. U.S. Dept Agr. Yearbook 1939, 1165 pp., illus.

Chapter 9

LUNGER DISEASE OF SHEEP

G.T. Creech[1]

[1] *G.T. Creech is Senior Veterinarian. Pathological Division. Bureau of Animal Industry.*

A chronic fatal disease has been known to exist among the sheep of Montana, Oregon, and other Northwestern States for a considerable time, the most prominent symptom of which is difficult or laboured breathing. Since this indicates that the lungs are affected, the disease is commonly referred to by herdsmen and sheep owners as lunger disease, and the affected animals are usually called lungers.

Marsh (4)[2], in Montana, who was among the first to make studies of this disease, found it to be of the nature of a chronic progressive pneumonia. He reported his findings in 1922. Later, rather extensive studies were also made by Creech and Gochenour (3), of the Bureau of Animal Industry.

A disease very similar in character, known as jagziekte, which has been recognized among the sheep of South Africa for many years, has been reported by Cowdry (*1*) and others. Because of the striking similarity of the lesions, or tissue injuries of jagziekte in South Africa and chronic progressive pneumonia in Montana, Cowdry and Marsh (2) made joint comparative studies of the two diseases and concluded that they were probably identical.

---

[2] Italic numbers in parentheses refer to Literature Cited.

Chronic progressive pneumonia is unquestionably of considerable economic importance. Marsh (*4*) estimated that the rate of loss from the disease among Montana sheep ranges from 2 to 10 percent, varying somewhat in different herds. The mortality among the animals affected is generally believed to be 100 percent. Observations have indicated that the losses are greater among older animals, but sheep of all ages appear to be susceptible.

Several theories as to the cause of this type of chronic pneumonia and jagziekte in sheep have been presented by different investigators. In his bacteriological studies of chronic progressive pneumonia, Marsh (*5*) frequently isolated a diphtheroid (a micro-organism closely resembling the diphtheria bacillus) and considered it a causative factor either associated with or secondary to certain other possible predis posing factors. Robertson (*7*), who was one of the earlier investigators of jagziekte in South African sheep, believed the causative factor in that disease was a protozoan. Mitchell (*6*) pointed to a specific virus as the cause of jagziekte. Cowdry and Marsh (*2*), in their later studies of the two diseases, reached the conclusion that although these chronic pneumonias, in which the lung lesions are particularly characteristic, may be due primarily to a specific cause, the disease complex as a whole is such as might be caused by a variety of predisposing and exciting factors operating over a period of time. In the investigations of the disease made in the Bureau of Animal Industry (*3*), extensive bacteriological studies of the lungs of affected sheep and various animal inoculations, or exposure tests, failed to reveal anything in the nature of a specific causative factor.

Since the disease occurs largely in range sheep, it seems rather probable that there may be certain predisposing environmental conditions, such as the methods of handling the sheep or irritation of the lung tissue by dust, which may make the animals more susceptible.

Symptoms and Control Measures

Because of the insidious nature of chronic progressive pneumonia of sheep, it is not known how long the animals may be affected before the first clinical symptoms can be observed. The first noticeable symptom is laboured breathing after exercise. As the disease progresses, there are more rapid respiration, dilated nostrils and flank breathing or pumping, even while the animal is at rest. More or less coughing and some nasal discharge have been observed in some cases. In the late stages the affected sheep show marked weakness and emaciation, and breathing becomes still more difficult. The disease eventually terminates in death.

No treatment for the disease is known. While there is no definite evidence to indicate that the disease is of an infectious or contagious nature, or that it may be transmitted from animal to animal, it would nevertheless seem advisable when the disease appears to separate the affected sheep from the healthy ones and, if practicable, to move the herd to an entirely new environment. The problem of controlling the disease by treatment or preventive measures will remain difficult of solution until more specific information is available about its cause.

A technical description of the conditions found on post mortem examination of sheep that have died of the disease follows.

Technical Description of Post Mortem Findings

The gross lesions found on autopsy are confined largely to the thoracic cavity. When the cavity is opened the lungs do not collapse but fill the entire cavity, and usually more or less fluid is found. Frequently extensive pleuritic adhesions are seen, and as a result of these fibrous proliferations the lung surface may show a constricted, or lobulated, appearance. In advanced cases there is extensive solidification of the lung tissue, which on cross sectioning has a characteristic pale or grayish appearance, with prominence of the lung lobules. In some cases a puslike material may be forced out of the bronchi and bronchioles, and occasionally bronchial concretions are observed. The associated bronchial and mediastinal lymph glands are swollen and moist, or edematous, in appearance.

The usual histological picture is that of a chronic catarrhal pneumonia. The walls of the alveoli show infiltrations of lymphocytes and large mononuclear cells. The cellular exudate in the alveoli consists of large mononuclear cells and leucocytes occasionally mixed with red cells. The large mononuclear cells in the lumen of the alveoli are frequently swollen and vacuolated.

Scattered through the affected lung tissue frequently are accumulations of lymphocytes, or lymphoid nodules, which have been referred to as tuberclelike nodules. Such nodules are seen in the peribronchial and also in the interalveolar tissue. In the consolidated portions of the lung tissue most of the alveoli are filled either with the cellular exudate or with mucous plugs. In some cases many of the alveoli and bronchioles are filled with polymorphonuclear leucocytes.

Epithelial proliferations of the alveoli and bronchioles, which are considered characteristic of progressive pneumonia, are observed in many cases of the disease. As the disease progresses, fibrous changes in the areas involved gradually increase, and in some cases practically complete fibrosis of a considerable portion of the lung tissue may be observed in the later stages.

Literature Cited

(1) COWDRY, E.V. (1925). STUDIES OF THE ETIOLOGY OF JAGZIEKTE. I. THE PRIMARY LESIONS. Jour. Expt. Med. 42: 323-333, illus.

(2) _____and MARSH, HADLEIGH (1927). COMPARATIVE PATHOLOGY OF SOUTH AFRICAN JAGZIEKTE AND MONTANA PROGRESSIVE PNEUMONIA OF SHEEP. Jour. Expt. Med. 45: 571-585, illus.

(3) CREECH, G.T., and GOCHENOUR, W.S. (1936). CHRONIC PROGRESSIVE PNEUMONIA OF SHEEP, WITH PARTICULAR REFERENCE TO ITS ETIOLOGY AND TRANSMISSION. Jour. Agr. Res. 52: 667-679, illus.

(4) MARSH, HADLEIGH (1923). PROGRESSIVE PNEUMONIA IN SHEEP. Amer. Vet. Med. Assoc. Jour. 62: 458-473.

(5) _____(1923). THE BACTERIOLOGY OF PROGRESSIVE PNEUMONIA OF SHEEP. Amer. Vet. Med. Assoc. Jour. 64: 304-317.

(6) MITCHELL, D.T. (1915). INVESTIGATIONS INTO JAGZIEKTE, OR CHRONIC CATARRHAL-PNEUMONIA OF SHEEP. Union So. Africa Dept. Agr. Dir. Res. Rpts. 8 and 4: [585]-614.

(7) ROBERTSON, WM. (1904). JAGZIEKTE OR CHRONIC CATARRHAL PNEUMONIA (SHEEP). Jour. Compar. Path. and Ther. 17: 221-224.

INDEX

S

T

V

W